Carryover Techniques

In Articulation and Phonological Therapy

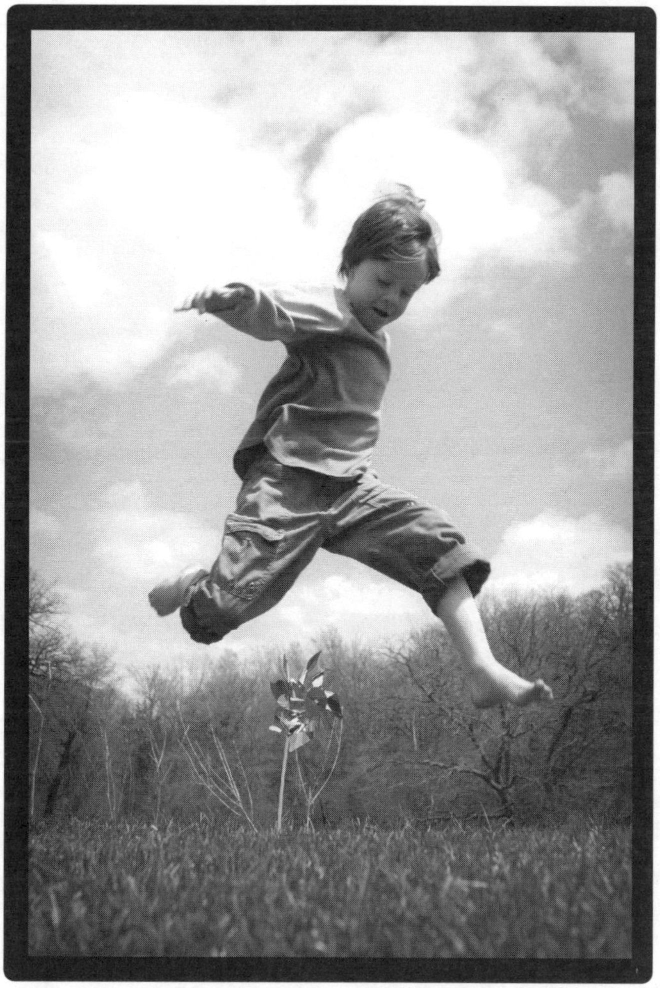

by Pam Marshalla, M.A., C.C.C.–SLP
Speech-Language Pathologist

Carryover Techniques in Articulation and Phonological Therapy

Printed in the United States

ISBN 978-0-9791749-3-3

Marshalla Speech & Language
Mill Creek, Washington, USA
www.pammarshalla.com

"Happy would be the lot of the speech-language pathologist if he [or she] did not have to worry about carryover."

– Elizabeth Bosley, 1981

Contents

Preface *vii*

Contributors *viii*

Editorial Notes *ix*

1. What is Carryover? 1
2. Research Studies on Generalization and Carryover 9
3. Managing the Carryover Process 21
4. Self-Monitoring for Carryover 31
5. Speech Production Activities for Carryover 49
6. The Role of Behavior Modification in Carryover 63
7. Conversational Speech in the Carryover Process 73
8. Personality, Emotion, and Attitude in Carryover 93
9. Games and Activities to Promote Carryover 109

Final Thoughts *151*

References *153*

Preface

Carryover is the term commonly used to refer to a client's ability to take an individual speech skill he has learned in the therapy room and to apply it broadly in all speaking situations. Many clients accomplish this task quickly and easily, but some do not. As a result, most speech-language pathologists struggle with the issue of carryover with one client or another at some point throughout their career. Direct attention to carryover cannot be neglected with these clients. Charles Van Riper, who is widely considered to be the Father of Articulation Therapy, said that carryover is one of the most important steps in the treatment of articulatory disorders. Carryover signals the completion of the articulation therapy process.

This is a book of ideas to ponder and use. It is not a research report, although research is reported in here. It also is not a cookbook of therapy techniques, although many recipes for treatment are contained herein. This book is intended to help practicing speech-language pathologists think through issues related to carryover so that they can design effective activities for clients in their charge. The contents have been gathered from five sources: (1) Research, (2) Historic textbooks on articulation therapy, (3) Modern textbooks on articulation and phonological therapy, (3) The author's three decades of clinical experience, and (4) Games and activities contributed by over 200 professional speech-language pathologists who responded to a request sent out via the publisher's website.

This book contains ideas, techniques, perspectives, insights, methods, procedures, games, and activities that researchers and practicing speech-language pathologists have found useful in the carryover process. This is a book written by a clinician for clinicians. It is meant to be a helpful aid to speech-language pathologists working with clients who are struggling with carryover. The author also hopes that the research community will use the methods discussed here as a source of ideas for future research projects.

Contributors

The following professional speech-language pathologists contributed ideas for this book. Hundreds of ideas were submitted and these were chosen because of their originality and pertinence to the topic. Pam Marshalla wishes to express her gratitude to these individuals for taking the time to gather and send their ideas. Contributors are listed with the page numbers on which their ideas appear.

Lisa Anderson *59*
Lynn-Rachel Ary *134*
Lindsey Baker *140*
Esther Baxter *141*
Renee Berg *123*
Gretchen Bergen *141*
Vivian Binnington *133*
Ricki Block *44*
Bonnie Chappell *146*
Robin Chopskie *144*
Leah Christianson *129*
Jennifer Code *44*
Susan Cohn *113*
Margaret Combs *86*
Lois B. Cook *112*
Denise Davis *114*
Kelly Davis *111*
Karen Dickson *57, 59*
Valerie Frost-McKinley *38*
Marti Fuller *38*
Paula Groothuis *132*
Linda Groszyk *140*
Linda Houge Gustafson *116*
Chana Hartman *45*
Shanna Hess *138*
Yoela Holman *44*
Sherri Hole *112*
Stacey R. Honowitz *124*
Melanie Hostetter *141*
Terri Jones *137*
Anne Kropf *141*
Alice Lamoreaux *145*
Amy Lang *120*
Karen Larssen *128*
Crystal Luk *134*
Judith Lunger-Bergh *133*
Cheryl Lunny *130*
Beth Marafiote *124*
Mollie Marlow *60*
Donna McDonough *128*
Grace Medina-Chow *128*
Mary Meehan *129*
Kim Metzgar *115*
Barbara Miller *111*
Stacey Misko *120*
Jane Moerman *116*
Debbie Neal *139*
Ellen Obrock *110*
Eliza Pelletreau *138*
Denise Prohaska *44*
Jill Richards *129*
Linda Richardson *44*
Donna Ridley *44, 142*
Alicia Roberts *119*
Janet Robinson *126*
Ann Roman *148*
Susan Freiman Ross *113*
Gailyn Walsh Ryan *110*
Zina Santos *127*
Shirley Schindeldecker *122*
June Schroeder *140*
Amy Schuchman *121*
Tamara Seeker *44*
Virginia Shawron *144*
Marybeth Shearron *139*
Philip Shively *38, 131*
LeAnn Sipple *137*
Kim Marty Smoot *127*
Nicole Spruill *112*
Sheila Stull *70, 139*
Mary Jane Thomas *113*
Anne Venables Eigner *114*
Kim Watson-Setliff *121*
Pamela Williams *143*
Jackie Zuelke-Karch *122*

Editorial Notes

It is understood that the term *speech-language pathologist* (SLP) is the title of the professional who is the subject of this book. This title will be used primarily. However, other titles are included in quoted material and elsewhere. The reader will discover terms such as *speech teacher, speech clinician, speech correctionist, speech therapist, clinician,* or *correctionist.* This has been done to add color to the text and to preserve the historical accuracy of quoted material.

Gender Designations

It is understood that clinicians and clients are represented by both genders. However, in this text, therapists generally are designated by female pronouns (*she, her, hers*) and clients generally are represented by male pronouns (*he, him, his*). Changes to this standard were used as needed. This designation has been applied simply to make the text less verbally cumbersome.

Traditional Articulation Therapy

We shall use the term *traditional articulation therapy* to refer to the process of articulation therapy outlined by Van Riper beginning with his publication of *Speech Correction: Principles and Methods* (1939).

English Language

This book is written in English for an English-speaking audience, and it concerns the North American English language. Application of this material to other languages can be expected but not assumed.

Alterations To Quoted Material

This text includes a variety of quoted material from other textbooks on articulation and phonology. The following editorial guidelines were employed:

- Minor alterations to punctuation were made to make older quotes more readable to today's audience. The original meaning of these statements was maintained.
- Grammatical errors used in quoted material were not corrected.
- Orthographic symbols were used instead of phonetic symbols in quoted material (see next).

Orthographic Symbols

Standard orthographic symbols have been employed instead of the International Phonetic Alphabet preferred by professional speech-language pathologists. This has been done so that parents, teachers, and other interested parties can read this material. Certain differences between phonemes were obliterated as a result. Specifically, /θ/ and /ð/ were treated as the same sound and symbolized as Th. Also, R is treated as a consonant only. The following orthographic symbol system was employed throughout the text.

Consonants

P – *pie*
B – *boy*
T – *toy*
D – *dog*
K – *car, key*
G – *go*

M – *moo*
N – *no*
Ng – *sing*

W – *we*
L – *low*
Y – *yes*
R – *row*

Th – *thumb, that*
F – *fee*
V – *vase*
S – *see*
Z – *zoo*
Sh – *shoe*
Zh – *beige*
Ch – *chew*
J – *jam*
H – *hat*

Vowels

uh – *up*
ee – *be*
oo – *too*
ah – *hot*
oh – *boat*

Chapter 1

What Is Carryover?

"Carryover might be said ... to be the 'eating' which is proof of the therapeutic 'pudding.'"

– Margaret Hall Powers, 1971

The word *carryover* is the term commonly used to refer to a client's ability to take an individual speech skill learned in the therapy room and to apply it broadly to all speaking situations. Articulation therapy is not over until carryover has been established, and carryover is only established when a client's new speech skill becomes customary in conversational speech. Some clients transfer their newly learned speech skills to conversation almost immediately and without effort. These are easy clients for whom we have to make almost no effort toward teaching carryover. But professional speech-language pathologists also treat clients who do not make this transfer well. These more difficult clients often need to be lead by the hand through all levels of therapy. They need to be carried through the carryover process, so to speak. They also need to be monitored regularly to make sure they are successful.

Carryover of articulation or phonological skills into real life speaking situations can be compared to acting. Reciting lines in a rehearsal hall is not all that actors must do. Eventually an actor must get on stage, or in front of a camera, to perform in front of others. Likewise, clients cannot just learn to articulate new phonemes correctly in the privacy of a therapy room. Eventually they must use their new skills with others out in the rest of their world. This is what we mean by carryover. This book discusses many aspects of carryover in articulation and phonological therapy. It is designed to help practicing speech-language pathologist think through the process in order to make clinical decisions about carryover activities for particular clients.

A Persistent Concern

Carryover has been a concern of speech-language pathologists since the inception of the profession, and it continues to be a stumbling block to the completion of a speech program for some clients even today. Consider the following statements about the importance of carryover made over the past 60 years:

- *1947*: "[Carryover is] one of the most important steps in the treatment of … articulatory … disorders" (Van Riper, 1947, p. 202).
- *1965*: "No child is able to watch his speech constantly and always incorporate the right sound into words. This process takes time" (Eisenson and Ogilvie, 1965, p. 247).
- *1971*: "It seems necessary in most cases to give specific and serious attention to promoting this carryover in order to ensure that it will take place" (Powers, 1971, p. 899).
- *1987*: "Unquestionably the greatest challenge facing clinicians of articulatory and phonological disorders today is the achievement of carryover" (Weiss, Gordon, and Lillywhite, 1987, p. 270).
- *1990*: "Carryover is a key to a child's success in speech and language therapy" (Hazel, 1990, p. 185).
- *1998*: "The ultimate goal of phonological intervention is the correct production of speech targets in spontaneous speech" (Ertmer and Ertmer, 1998, p. 67).
- *2004*: "Generalization [as an aspect of carryover] is a critical and all-important step in the learning process for all children who receive treatment for phonologic disorders" (Bernthal and Bankson, 2004, p. 275).

Who's To Blame?

It is easy to blame the client when carryover is incomplete. Lack of carryover can make a client appear forgetful, immature, stubborn, spacey, unintelligent, or uncooperative. Complaints are made that these clients could complete their articulation programs if they simply tried harder. But trying harder is not necessarily the solution. Students who have difficulty with carryover simply are demonstrating that they need careful guidance in this area, a fact that makes this aspect of therapy no different than any other. Carryover simply is part of therapy. Some clients need very little guidance in carryover and others need to be led by the hand.

Changes In Time

Carryover approaches change as therapy programs progress over time. At first, carryover is controlled, disciplined, carefully measured, regulated, and kept in check. Over time carryover becomes automatic and it is done without conscious thought, without the need to make a decision, and without intention. The final stages of carryover involve spontaneous speech, or speech that arises from natural impulses rather than from planning or suggestion. Completing the carryover process requires that new speech skills are used habitually, regularly, repetitively, and unconsciously. Ultimately carryover will become unrestrained and uninhibited. This is the standard view of carryover summarized neatly by two of our earliest writers: "Develop the patient's tentative and uncertain production of the new sound into a firmly rooted speech habit, [and] transform it from a consciously performed into an automatic act" (Borden and Busse, 1925, p. 187).

Generalization

The terms *carryover* and *generalization* often are used interchangeably. "[Generalization] is the principle that learning one behavior in a particular environment often carries over to other similar behaviors, environments, or untrained contexts" (Bernthal and Bankson, 2004, p. 275). This means that the client takes his new articulation or phonological skill and uses it in other linguistic, phonetic, phonological, semantic, syntactic, pragmatic, and situational contents. Generalization is the essence of carryover, and generalization is the thing that easy clients do automatically. Consider the acquisition of any phoneme. At first the phoneme is learned alone or in a syllable. To generalize means to begin to use the phoneme:

- IN ALL TYPES OF WORDS: Nouns, main verbs, secondary verbs, adjectives, adverbs, conjunctions, articles, negatives, and sound expressions (e.g., *wow!*).
- IN ALL WORD POSITIONS: Initial, medial, final, and blends.
- IN WORDS OF ANY LENGTH: Words of one syllable, two syllables, three syllables, and so forth.
- AS BOTH A PHONEME AND A MORPHEME WHERE APPLICABLE: For example, S is also used as a plural morpheme (*cats*); a possessive morpheme (*cat's paw*); a third person regular tense verb marker (*The cat walks.*); the auxiliary form of to be (*The cat's purring.*); and the copula form of to be (*The cat's big.*).
- IN WORDS USED IN ALL MANNER OF SPOKEN LITERATURE: Songs, stories, poems, paragraphs, rhymes, raps, and so forth.
- IN WORDS SPOKEN FOR A VARIETY OF PRAGMATIC PURPOSES: Stating, requesting, asking, answering, accepting, denying, demanding, pleading, refusing, informing, instructing, questioning, and so forth.
- WHEN SPEAKING WORDS TO ALL COMMUNICATION PARTNERS: Parents, siblings, teachers, peers, and so forth.
- WHEN SPEAKING IN ALL LOCATIONS AND SITUATIONS: At home, school, on the playground, in the car, on the bus, at the grocery store, and so forth.

Overgeneralization: A Clumsy Beginning to Carryover

The process of articulation and phonological therapy often results in *overgeneralization*, or the process of taking generalization too far. A client overgeneralizes when he uses a target speech skill more often and for more purposes than necessary. For example, it is common for young children to overgeneralize stridency. A child who has been saying *Christmas tree* as "Kee-Muh-Tee" may change it to "Shee-Shuh-Shee" once he gains stridency and begins to overgeneralize it.

Most writers in the area of phonology seem to consider overgeneralization a problem that needs remediation. But I consider overgeneralization to be a beneficial skill because it signals a clumsy beginning to the generalization or carryover process. In fact, I actually like and encourage overgeneralization in my therapy because I consider it a stage of development. Overgeneralization reveals that a client is experimenting broadly with the phoneme, feature, or process that has been acquired. Overgeneralization is like a new toy that a child has been given and simply cannot put down. Most children are driven to play with a new toy exclusively for a very concentrated period as they figure out just how many ways there are to use it. They *over-play* with a new toy. After a while, however, they soften this exclusive interest and integrate the new toy into the existing set of old toys.

My clinical experiences have taught me that the over-use of a new speech skill may dominate for a while but, like a new toy, this excessive preoccupation with the new speech skill usually fades with time. Occasionally a client does not outgrow his over-use of his new skill and he must be taught how to stop doing it, although I suspect that this is a rare phenomenon. In more than three decades of therapy where I served literally thousands of clients, I found it necessary to help only a few clients stop overgeneralizing. Most clients seem to stop overgeneralizing when given more time to develop a discriminative use of their new skill.

Transfer

Carryover also can involve *transfer* of skill from one phoneme to another, a process that can occur automatically or can be taught. For example, if a client can close his lips to say B, we can use B to teach him how to say other phonemes that require lip closure, namely P and M. Essentially we are transferring the lip closing feature from one phoneme to another. This transfer process also has been called *across-sound generalization* and *across-feature generalization*. In general, the easy client usually makes these transfers automatically while the difficult client may not.

Maintenance

Another aspect of carryover is *maintenance* defined as "the continued use of the target sound in all speaking situations over time" (Weiss, Gordon, and Lillywhite, 1987, p. 277). We are speaking of the time in treatment when the client is expected to maintain his skill level while he is gradually faded away from weekly therapy. The client's treatment sessions might be reduced from once per week to once per month, to once per three months, to once per six months, and so forth. The purpose of these continuing sessions is to make sure that the client is maintaining top performance without weekly instruction.

Maintenance sessions do not have to be formal treatment lessons. In the modern public school setting, maintenance often is checked simply by seeking out the client and speaking with him informally for a few minutes. This can take place in the hall, in the cafeteria, on the playground, in an assembly, or in any other convenient meeting place in the school. In the private clinic, maintenance sessions can take place in the office, or they can take place via phone, or on-line video phoning, so that travel time can be eliminated. Easy clients maintain their skills and usually can terminate therapy quickly and easily. Difficult clients may need a long period of monitored maintenance.

Changing Habits

To establish a new speech habit means to break an old one. Breaking an old habit and gaining a new one can be difficult. Have you ever tried to break a habit like smoking, overeating, or twirling your hair? Have you ever tried to gain a new habit like walking every day, paying bills on time, or reading instead of watching television every evening? Changing habits is difficult to do. Humans like to be comfortable, and changing habits makes us uncomfortable for a while. In addition, sometimes we simply forget that we were supposed to be changing habits. For example, have you ever realized in April that you forgot about a New Year's resolution made in January? Breaking an old habit, and acquiring a new one, takes awareness, memory, willingness, determination, persistence, and conscious control. The speech-language pathologist's job is to figure out how to stimulate these qualities in clients who display poor carryover. The SLP often plays the role of teacher, counselor, coach, and friend to clients struggling in this process. The ability to take control of a changing habit often differentiates an easy client from a difficult one. Easy clients change habits quickly and easily while difficult clients do not. Van Riper perhaps said it best: "New habits must be taught and old ones broken. People differ in their modifiability" (Van Riper, 1949, p. 29).

Carryover Is Not...

We should say a few words about what carryover is not. Carryover is not extra work tagged on to the end of an articulation or phonological program. Carryover is not something clients should have to figure out on their own. Carryover is not constant drill, although a certain amount of drill can assist in the carryover process. Carryover does not mean to persistently remind a client to speak correctly, and it does not mean to correct a client every time he makes an error. Again, Van Riper: "No one can watch himself all the time, and we all hate to be nagged" (Van Riper, 1949, p. 204).

Perhaps most importantly today, we must state clearly that carryover is not reading out loud. Reading aloud can be employed as a method of carryover as we shall discuss later. But reading out loud is not the final product of carryover. Even our earliest clinicians understood that reading out loud and speaking spontaneously were two completely different processes: "Reading aloud is an essentially different process from repeating words or from spontaneous speech" (Blanton and Blanton, 1919, p. 192).

How are reading aloud and spontaneous speaking different? Reading is slower and more methodical than spontaneous speech. In reading, one is focused on the task of reading the words already written out, while speaking involves newly generated ideas that come directly from the heart and mind. Carryover involves speaking correctly under all spontaneous speaking conditions, while reading is not spontaneous and it only represents one type of speaking. Some clients are perfectly able to use correct articulation while reading out loud, yet cannot maintain correct speech in spontaneous conversation. For these reasons reading can be used as a carryover technique, but it cannot be considered the final product. Most therapists seem to consider reading as a bridge from single words to conversation. The stimulation of carryover probably will involve reading for those clients who can read, but carryover itself involves much more than that.

Ranking Carryover Methods

In 1980, Polson published the results of a research project in which 125 practicing public school speech-language pathologists were asked to rank the order of effectiveness of twelve carryover methods. The order in which therapists found these carryover methods to be effective were ranked as follows, from those they found most effective to those they considered least effective:

1. Self-monitoring (most effective)
2. Practice or drill until performance is automatic
3. Emphasis on a structured behavior modification system
4. Practice with people outside of therapy

5. Working outside the clinic with the therapist
6. Auditory discrimination training
7. Homework assignments
8. Reminders to be used in the outside world
9. Creative drama
10. Integration of the articulation work into the language arts program
11. Client-designed homework assignments
12. Practice under various emotional conditions (least effective)

It is interesting to note that these practicing speech-language pathologists thought that the three most important things to assure carryover were to help the client learn to pay attention to his own speech, to make him practice or drill, and to use a consistent reward and punishment system as the client rehearses his new speech skill. It is also interesting to note that these therapists considered the integration of articulation work into the language arts program — what we would call the *literacy* model today — to be one of the three least effective methods of carryover for articulation.

No Perfect Technique

Most speech-language pathologists today probably would agree that there is no single correct or best carryover technique. Certainly there are none that have been proven to work in all cases. Carryover techniques are designed for the individual client and are selected with a variety of perspectives in mind:

- The client's chronological age, cognitive status, language level, hearing ability, and motor coordination need consideration.
- The personality, learning style, and interests of the client and the therapist also shape the carryover process.
- The schedule of therapy, size of the group, materials at hand, and employment setting play important roles in the selection of carryover activities.
- Carryover procedures are adjusted according to whether or not parents, caregivers, teachers, siblings, peers, or others participate in the process.
- Carryover techniques are chosen when they prove beneficial to the client at hand. This is the most important factor of them all.

Lack of Carryover

Carryover can fail for many reasons, each reason as individual as the client who is failing. Often there is a combination of reasons for failure. I am reminded of an e-mail sent to me by a practicing speech-language pathologist whose elementary-age client failed to carryover his newly learned R phoneme. The SLP wrote that he had done quite well in therapy, and that she had gotten him to the point at which he could read word lists with correct R when given cues from the therapist. The client was dismissed from therapy at that point. Re-testing one year later revealed that the client's R was still incorrect. Most experienced therapists would agree that this client's lack of carryover could be due to any one of several important factors. For example:

1. The ability to read word lists correctly does not indicate that the client has control over his new production at any other level. The client will need to work on the more advanced levels of production — phrases, sentences, paragraphs, and conversation.
2. The ability to read words from a list does not suggest that the client has made a routine of his new speech skill. Activities must be employed to make his target habitual.
3. A client's ability to produce correct phonemes in words does not mean he understands why this work is important to his life. The ability to produce a phoneme in a new correct way needs to be important to the client or he may lose it shortly after therapy is terminated.
4. A client's ability to say his target correctly does not mean that he is monitoring himself. Clients must be taught to self-monitor in order to take them through the carryover process.
5. A client's ability to perform well with one person in a therapy room does not mean he is willing and able to perform well with other people in other situations.
6. A client who is relying on cues must be taught not to rely on them. Cues usually have to be faded before a client can be dismissed from regular treatment.
7. A client's carryover program cannot be left to chance. More direct intervention is necessary in many cases.
8. Therapy follow-up must take place sooner than one year so that clients can be reinstated if they are failing.

*

Chapter 1 Summary

What Is Carryover?

- Carryover is the term commonly used to refer to a client's ability to take an individual speech skill learned in the therapy room and to apply it broadly in all speaking situations.
- Carryover can be automatic for some children, but it can be a stumbling block for others.
- Carryover approaches change as therapy progresses over time.
- The terms carryover and generalization often are used interchangeably.
- Carryover can involve the transfer of skill from one phoneme to another.
- Overgeneralization is the process of taking generalization too far. Overgeneralization may be the first sign of carryover. It can serve as a clumsy beginning to the carryover process.
- Carryover also involves maintenance, or the ability to maintain skill level while gradually fading away from weekly therapy.
- Carryover involves habit breaking. Breaking an old habit and acquiring a new one takes awareness, memory, willingness, determination, persistence, and conscious control.
- Carryover is not extra work, constant drill, persistent reminding, relentless correction, or reading aloud.
- Techniques that practicing therapists have judged as being the most effective to the development of carryover skill include self-monitoring, practice, and emphasis on a structured behavior modification system.
- Techniques that practicing therapists judged as being the least effective to the development of carryover skill include integration of articulation work in the language arts program, homework activities of the client's own design, and practice under various emotional conditions.
- There does not seem to be any one correct or best carryover technique. Instead there are many from which to choose and match to individual clients.
- Monitoring carryover needs to be a process of observing conversational speech.
- Lack of carryover can be due to any one of several important factors.

Chapter 2

Research Studies on Generalization and Carryover

"We always have sought to base our decisions and actions on the best possible evidence."

– David Sackett, Scott Richardson
William Rosenberg, and Brian Haynes, 1997

This chapter summarizes research in regard to carryover. A few studies specifically on carryover have been undertaken in modern times. Studies on aspects of generalization are more prevalent than those on carryover itself, and they comprise the bulk of this chapter. Before we review the literature, however, let us say a few words about the *evidence-based practice*, the *practicality of therapy*, and *four practical approaches* to treatment utilized by our predecessors.

The Evidence-Based Practice

The modern speech-language pathologist recognizes the challenge to place carryover techniques within the scope of the *evidence-based practice* (EBP). The American Speech-Language-Hearing Association (ASHA) has defined the goal of the EBP as follows:

> *"The goal of EBP is the integration of clinical expertise, best current evidence, and client values to provide high-quality services reflecting the interests, values, needs, and choices of the individuals we serve"* (ASHA, 2010).

Following ASHA, speech-language pathologists create an evidence-based practice by integrating evidence from three sources: the lab, the clinic, and the client. As a result, some methods of carryover are adapted from the results of formal research (the lab), others come from the therapist's prior clinical experiences (the clinic), and still others arise from working with the client himself (the client). Practicing speech-language pathologists integrate carryover ideas from these three sources to comply with the demands of the EBP in their clinical work. Following ASHA's guideline, the ideas for this book have been gathered from both scientific research and the experiences of practicing therapists.

The Practicality of Therapy

It is important to recognize the practical nature of the EBP. David Sackett and his colleagues, the physicians who first defined the EBP, said that laboratory evidence, or *external evidence*, by itself does not create an effective therapy program: "External clinical evidence can inform, but can never replace, individual clinical expertise" (Sackett et al, 1997, p. 3-4). Sackett and his colleagues were saying that the evidence that comes from laboratory research is not enough to carry out clinical practice. They were saying that the EBP integrates laboratory evidence together with the evidence one has gained from working directly with patients.

The speech-language pathologist's job is not to replicate research projects. In fact, speech-language pathologists modify and experiment with researched methods in order to discover the value a particular method may hold for a particular client. Therapists purposefully alter researched methods to suit the immediate needs of the client at hand. They also make up their own methods based upon basic scientific knowledge. The speech-language pathologist's work is to discover which methods of treatment prove beneficial to the particular client at hand, and we often select methods regardless of laboratory evidence. If a tried method results in positive changes for a particular client, then it is valuable because it reflects the client's interests, values, needs, choices, and skills. Effective methods are continued while ineffective ones are discontinued. Such is the practical and realistic nature of the evidence-based practice.

> *"Making good clinical decisions is not easy. The existence of high-quality research can certainly help inform clinical decisions, but research is just one of several factors that influence clinical decisions. Additional factors are the two other components of EBP — client values and clinical expertise — as well as a clinician's theoretical perspective, service delivery considerations, the opinion of experts, and experimental validation with individual clients"* (Kamhi, 2006, p. 277).

Four Classic Concepts

Throughout the history of therapeutic enterprises, theoreticians and therapists alike have discussed four concepts that seem to have gone out of favor recently in our zeal to provide evidence for everything done in therapy. These are the *working theory,* the process of *trial-and-error*, the use of *common sense*, and a teacher's *natural teaching ability*. These ideas used to be cornerstones of all educational and therapeutic discussions, and they were written about in virtually all textbooks on traditional articulation therapy. But they are disappearing from modern evidence-driven texts. We shall discuss each briefly because these ideas are still relevant in today's evidence-based practice.

Working Theories

A *working theory* is a hypothesis, a premise, a presumption, or a guess about a treatment approach that one can assume is true until it is proven otherwise. For example, most practicing therapists recognize that success in articulation therapy is more assured if clients periodically watch themselves perform in a mirror. This idea has been discussed time and again in textbooks on articulation therapy. However, we have no direct proof of the effectiveness of mirrors because no one has bothered to study this simple idea in populations of children with articulation error. Using a mirror for speech training is a working theory that can continue to be used until formal research disproves it. Working theories form the basis of many carryover procedures used by practicing speech-language pathologists. We have included therapy ideas based on working theories all throughout this book. Working theories build one's clinical experiences in the evidence-based practice.

Trial-and-Error

Old-time writers of articulation therapy virtually always discussed *trial-and-error* in therapy. Trial-and-error is a process that unfolds in three stages: (1) A therapist tries a method to see if it works with a particular client, (2) The therapist continues to use the method if it proves effective with that client, and (3) The therapist discontinues or changes the method if it proves ineffective with that client. This is what therapists do every single day. Thus, even if there are piles of evidence indicating that a certain method is effective with a group of research subjects, each SLP still has to determine if that method is effective for the individual client at hand. We use trial-and-error to do this. We also use trial-and-error to see if a method that proved effective the last time we worked with our client still helps him today. Methods that trial-and-error prove to be ineffective are altered, abandoned, or held in reserve for another time. Trial-and-error is the process that builds one's clinical expertise in an evidence-based practice. Trial-and-error is the process clinicians use to discover the needs, desires, values, and preferences of individual clients.

Common Sense

The practicing speech-language pathologist often has nothing but *common sense* upon which to make therapeutic decisions. Common sense is the natural intelligence that develops through observation of everyday life experiences. Common sense must be employed when therapists discover that there is simply no evidence in regard to a particular topic, and when they have never seen a particular problem before. For example, common sense dictates that children will carryover new articulation skills better if they don't spend all their free time engaged in on-line social networking. Our common sense tells us this must be true, because if a client is on-line during all of his unstructured time, then he is affording himself no opportunities to practice his new speech skill with others. Common sense dictates that the client needs to walk away from the computer on occasion to interact with others. Do we have any proof that decreasing time on the computer enhances carryover? No. This simply is common sense at work. There are numerous processes of remediation that therapists just *know*, and many of these come from common sense. Common sense is not a trivial matter, and it should not be dismissed in our fervor for laboratory evidence. Common sense should rule at all times during the treatment process. Many ideas presented in this book arose from simple common sense. Common sense is fundamental to the development of the clinical expertise demanded of the evidence-based practice.

Natural Teaching Ability

Traditional therapists often wrote about the need to use one's *natural teaching ability* to be an effective clinician. The natural teaching ability is the talent, aptitude, flair, faculty, endowment, or gift one brings to the therapeutic process. Most speech-language pathologists have a natural teaching ability. In fact, it probably was that very ability that drove most of us into the field in the first place. Unfortunately, the idea of giftedness seems out of step with the new evidence-based thrust, but one's natural teaching ability cannot be ignored in the therapeutic setting. It is part of our clinical expertise. Our natural teaching ability allows us to face a difficult client, for whom we have no idea what to do, and to figure out what to do right on the spot. Our affinity for teaching allows us to observe carefully and to design useful teaching activities that no one has thought of before. We are teachers of speech correction. Those of us with the gift of teaching often can figure out what needs to be done to get ideas across to students quite easily, regardless of whether there is any research that has proven that the idea will work. Just like common sense, one's natural teaching ability is not a trivial matter. One's natural teaching ability must rule the day when there is very little evidence, and this is the case in regard to carryover.

> *"The skilled practitioner is resourceful in adapting methods to needs ... there is no substitute for creative imagination in planning teaching activities of any kind"* (Carrell, 1968, p. 92–102).

Research Findings

The rest of this chapter is devoted to a review of the literature relevant to carryover and generalization in articulation and phonological therapy. I always have found the process of reading through a review of pertinent research to be a laborious process, so I have taken the liberty of presenting this material in a different way for easier access. Studies are arranged by topics, topic areas have been arranged alphabetically, and the studies within each topic are presented as bulleted items arranged chronologically so the reader can see the evolution of ideas over time. A simple one-line description summarizes each study's findings in regard to carryover. It is recognized that each of these studies demonstrated far more than the tidbits offered here. I have attempted to focus only on the one or two pieces of information per article that have the most relevance to our topic. Readers are referred to the original articles to gain a better perspective of each project's scope of study.

Across-Language Generalization

At least two studies have indicated that generalization of a phoneme can occur from one language to another.

- McNutt (1994) ascertained that training correct S in English can generalize to a correct production of S in French.
- Ray (2002) demonstrated that generalization can occur across three languages when a cognitive-linguistic approach and minimal pairs are used.

Behavior Modification and Carryover

Some investigators have been interested in the relationship between behavior modification, speech contracts, dismissal criteria, and reward systems in the carryover process.

- Winitz and Bellerose (1963) suggested that phoneme generalization can be maintained with reinforcement.
- Wing and Heimgartner (1973) demonstrated that five levels of treatment could be effective in the carryover process: (1) oral reading, (2) oral reading and oral discussion, (3) structured conversation within a time span and with a pre-selected topic, (4) unstructured conversation with an increased time span, and (5) unstructured conversation within an extended time span.
- Diedrich and Bangert (1976) studied clients who were dismissed from therapy after having achieved 75% correct criteria for production of S and R in word lists and in conversation. They found that these clients retained articulation skill as well as clients who were kept in therapy longer.
- Polson (1980) studied the opinions of professional speech-language pathologists in regard to carryover. Consistent behavior modification was ranked as the third most important element of twelve carryover methods.
- Tabor and Hambrecht (1997) found an increase in S productions by students who signed contracts and received rewards for meeting their contract standards. However, clients reverted to previous poor levels of performance when contracts were finished. The authors suggested that contracts should involve a longer time period and that rewards should be more valuable to the client (they used rewards costing under $2.00).

Distinctive Features and Generalization

A number of studies have indicated that training a distinctive feature in one phoneme can stimulate production of another phoneme that utilizes the same feature.

- Winitz and Bellerose (1963) demonstrated that the similarity of phonetic features effects phoneme generalization in positive ways.
- McReynolds and Bennett (1972) revealed that subjects could generalize phonological features [+strident], [+voice], and [+continuant] to many phonemes when only one phoneme was taught.
- Costello and Onstein (1976) found that distinctive features could generalize from one phoneme to another.
- Rosenwinkel (1976) demonstrated that generalization of [+strident] to other phonemes occurred when S was targeted.
- Weiner (1981) reported that final fricatives could be stimulated by training word-final stops when minimal pairs were used.
- Dunn and Till (1982) determined that distinctive features can transfer from one phoneme to another.
- Dinnsen and Elbert (1984) demonstrated that therapy focused on training sounds for which the client had the least amount of phonological knowledge resulted in the widest generalization.
- Powell and Elbert (1984) revealed that children can generalize phonological targets.
- Monahan (1986) revealed that common phonological patterns can generalize from trained to untrained words in children with multiple misarticulations.
- Zagar and Locke (1986) demonstrated that manner and voice features generalized more easily to untrained words than did the place feature. The authors speculated that per-

haps there are children who are *manner-cued* and those that are *place-cued.*

- Dinnsen, Chin, Elbert, and Powell (1990) revealed that generalization to phonetically less complex sounds could occur when phonetically more complex sounds were taught.
- Williams (1991) indicated that speech is improved when a new class of phonemes enters the phonological system, even though the full set of phonemes within that class is not completely organized and errors still occur.

Imitation Versus Spontaneous Productions in Generalization

Two studies have investigated the generalization that occurs on imitation tasks versus spontaneous speech tasks.

- Wright, Shelton and Arndt (1969) disclosed that subjects generalized better when imitative tasks were used.
- Diedrich and Bangert (1980) suggested that generalization in older school-age children occurred equally well on imitative and spontaneous tasks.

Limitations of Generalization

Some studies have indicated that generalization may not occur in some populations.

- Sommers et al (1970) demonstrated that children with cognitive skills in the educable range were unable to carry correct phoneme productions over to novel situations. They suggested that these children might need special focus and an on-going effort directed toward carryover.
- Raymore and McLean (1972) found that word-position generalization may not occur in children with mental retardation.
- Rockman and Elbert (1982) revealed that word-position generalization may not occur in children with severely restricted phonetic inventories.
- Zagar and Locke (1986) suggested that limitations in cognitive skill affect children's ability to generalize phonetic features.

Number of Exemplars and Generalization

Several investigators have studied the relationship between the number of words trained and generalization.

- Costello and Bosler (1976) found that more generalization to new environments occurred when more word varieties were trained.
- Elbert and McReynolds (1978) established that generalization can occur with only a small number of exemplars.
- Monahan (1986) showed that generalization of phonological processes can occur with a minimal number of training stimuli.
- Elbert, Powell, and Swartzlander (1991) demonstrated that only a small number of minimal pairs could promote generalization, although their subjects showed wide variability in this skill.

Parents, Peers, Teachers, Aids and Carryover

Several studies have revealed that progress in articulation and phonological skills can be made when parents, peers, teachers, or teacher aids are involved in the training process.

- Sommers et al (1959) suggested that more rapid improvement in articulation may occur when parents are involved.
- Marquardt (1959) described a successful carryover program called *Speech Pals* in which other children were being used to encourage carryover. The Speech Pals attended therapy with the client, and then they listened to him read aloud in the classroom every day.
- Sommers (1962) demonstrated that subjects whose mothers were trained to assist in the correction of misarticulations made significantly greater improvement than subjects whose mothers were not trained.
- Engel et al (1966) suggested that college roommates, fraternity and sorority members, and siblings could help in the carryover process.
- Mowrer, Baker, and Schultz (1968) demonstrated positive results in articulation therapy when parents were involved in treatment.
- Carrier (1970) found that children whose parents were involved in treatment scored higher post-treatment than those with minimal parent involvement.
- Bankson and Byrne (1972) found that conversational proficiency in the home reflected that found in the clinic.
- Wing and Heimgartner (1973) reported that parents could be used effectively in their carryover program.
- Engel and Groth (1976) demonstrated that teacher aids can be helpful in the carryover process.
- Hazel (1990) suggested that a peer homework monitoring system could be effective in the carryover process.

Phoneme Selection and Generalization

Investigators have studied the relationship between phonemes that were taught and those that were not taught.

- Elbert, Shelton and Arndt (1967) disclosed that training one phoneme could generalize to another.
- Leonard and Webb (1971) found a significant carryover of correct production from trained to untrained words, although performance on the actual practice words was higher.
- Elbert, Dinneson, and Powell (1984) revealed that training fricatives enhances the learning of stop consonants.
- Young (1987) found that weak syllables and consonant clusters could generalize from trained to untrained words.
- Gierut, Morrisette, Hughes, and Rowland (1996) found that clients could acquire early-developing sounds when later-developing sounds were taught, but that the reverse was not true.

Phonological Knowledge and Generalization

Several studies have indicated that general phonological knowledge can affect generalization.

- Dinnsen and Elbert (1984) found that productive phonologic knowledge influences generalization.
- Elbert and Gierut (1986) also found that productive phonologic knowledge influences generalization.
- Gierut, Elbert and Dinnsen (1987) demonstrated that greater generalization occurs when children have more information about phonemes.
- Gierut (1989) also found that productive phonologic knowledge influences generalization when word-initial position consonants were trained.

Practice and Generalization

Investigators have been interested in the relationship between the amount and type of practice necessary for generalization and carryover to occur.

- Bankson and Byrne (1972) found that overpractice can be somewhat effective as a method of carryover.
- Bankson and Byrne (1972) showed that motor-based treatment approaches can facilitate generalization of phonemes to conversation.
- Bankson and Byrne (1972) found that a target sound carried over to conversational speech at home and in the clinic after rapid word list training.
- Elbert and McReynolds (1978) found that the amount of training was an important variable in generalization.
- Diedrich and Byrne (1980) found that 50% of their study subjects generalized /s/ and /z/ immediately, suggesting that clinicians may want to start carryover programming early in treatment.
- Polson (1980) found that practice was judged by professional speech-language pathologists to be the second most important of twelve elements for successful carryover.
- Gierut, Elbert, and Dinnsen (1987) found that the greatest amount of generalization occurs when practice is included in therapy.
- Elbert, Dinnsen, Swartzlander, and Chin (1990) found that many children do generalize correct sound production to conversational speech without direct treatment on conversational speech.
- Powell, Elbert, and Dinnsen (1991) reported that learning a target sound can occur even when we try to teach another phoneme for which the client is not stimulable.
- Kamhi (2000) found that practice and functional communication work together. They do not need to be viewed as antagonists in carryover: "Instead, practice should be viewed as an effective way to facilitate productive use of speech and language forms in meaningful communicative situations" (p. 185).

Self-Monitoring and Carryover

Many studies have indicated that self-monitoring techniques can facilitate situational carryover.

- Diedrich (1971) revealed that charting progress was an effective tool in self-monitoring during the carryover process.
- Engel and Groth (1976) demonstrated that hand-raising can be an effective tool in self-monitoring during the carryover process.
- Ruscello and Shelton (1979) found that children generalize better when they use three processes—when they mentally plan out their articulatory movements, then produce targets, and then assess their own productions. Children who produced targets without mental planning and self-evaluation performed less well.
- Polson (1980) discovered that auditory self-monitoring was judged by professional speech-language pathologists to be the most important of twelve elements for successful carryover.
- Koegel, Koegel, and Ingham (1986) also demonstrated that hand-raising can be an effective tool in self-monitoring during the carryover process.
- Shriberg and Kwiatkowski (1987) ascertained that self-monitoring was more important than auditory bombardment, auditory discrimination, and minimal contrast training in facilitating carryover to spontaneous speech.
- Koegel, Koegel, Van Voy, and Ingham (1988) reported that children taught how to monitor their conversational speech outside of the therapy room carryover S and Z better than when they are taught to monitor in the clinic.
- Shriberg and Kwiatkowski (1990) indicated that awareness of speech sounds is best trained by working on the sounds themselves in production activities.
- Gray and Shelton (1992) tried to replicate Koegel et at (1988), but they achieved different results. They reported that the ability to self-monitor accurately within the clinic did *not* appear to affect carryover positively. The authors attributed their poorer results in carryover to the following: Too many therapy conditions, too many different therapists per client, too few self-monitoring requirements, a shorter period of treatment, and tasks that were more complex.

Setting and Generalization

Two studies have looked at the relationship between the training setting and generalization.

- Costello and Bosler (1976) demonstrated that situational generalization can be facilitated, although no one setting in their study enhanced carryover more than another. They also found that the physical dimensions of the room did not influence articulation performance in their carryover process.
- Irwin, Weston, Griffith, and Rocconi (1976) demonstrated that the paired stimuli approach can be an effective tool in generalizing phonemes trained in the therapy room to other non-experimental settings.

Syllables, Nonsense Material, Error Productions, and Generalization

Several studies have investigated whether training on nonsense syllables can generalize to real words.

- Powell and McReynolds (1969) found that practice of nonsense words can generalize to real words.
- Leonard and Webb (1971) found that training a client to listen to correct productions as well as error productions facilitated correct phoneme production and carryover of the target.
- Costello and Onstine (1976) showed that practice of nonsense words generalized to real words.
- Elbert and McReynolds (1978) found that several different syllable shapes have an equal effect on generalization. They studied CV, VC, CCV, and CVCC, and a variety of vowels.
- Gierut, Morrisette, and Ziemer (2010) demonstrated that nonwords induced greater, more rapid system-wide generalization as a function of treatment than did real words in children with phonological impairment. Children who were exposed to nonwords maintained their high levels of performance even after treatment was withdrawn.

Word-Position and Generalization

Many studies have revealed that generalization can occur from one word position to another.

- Powell and McReynolds (1969) reported that generalization can occur across word positions.
- Zehel, Shelton, Arndt, Wright, and Elbert (1972) demonstrated that generalization can occur across word positions when S is trained.
- Elbert and McReynolds (1975) demonstrated that generalization can occur across word positions although success can vary between clients.
- Ruscello (1975) determined that better generalization of phonemes occurred when three positions were trained — initial, medial, and final. Less generalization occurred when only one position was trained, although some clients were able to make word position generalizations when only one position was trained.
- Olswang and Bain (1985) established that generalization of S from one word position to another could occur. They also found that L did not generalize from initial to final position.
- Weaver-Spurlock and Brasseur (1988) indicated that S can generalize from one word position to another.
- Wolfe, Blocker, and Prater (1988) suggested that generalization may be more effective when inflection is added to targets.
- Miccio and Ingrisano (2000) demonstrated in a case study that fricatives taught in the initial position can generalize to words with the target in other positions, and they can generalize to connected speech.

Additional Sources

The following references are good additional sources on research related to carryover and generalization:

- TEXTBOOK: The text, *Articulation and Phonological Disorders* by Bernthal and Bankson (2004), contains an excellent discussion of research in the areas of generalization and carryover in articulation and phonological therapy. (See pp. 275-289).
- TUTORIAL: An article entitled "Constructivist strategies in phonological intervention: Facilitating self-regulation for carryover" by Ertmer and Ertmer (1998), is a good modern-day journal tutorial on carryover. They review the literature and discuss carryover in light of learning theories, selecting phonological strategies, self-regulation, constructivism, increasing motivation, and so forth.
- CASE STUDY: An article entitled "Planning for phonological generalization: An approach to treatment target selection" by Powell (1991) is a clinical focus article in which the authors present their process of planning phoneme generalization for one five-year-old child with multiple misarticulations and high unintelligibility. Phoneme selection, planning procedures, and their effect on generalization, are described.
- TEXTBOOK: The text, *Clinical Management of Articulatory and Phonological Disorders* by Curtis Weiss, Mary Gordon, and Herald Lillywhite (1987), contains an excellent chapter on carryover.

*

Chapter 2 Summary

Research Studies on Generalization and Carryover

- Carryover techniques must be placed within the parameters of an evidence-based practice (EBP).
- Evidence for the EBP comes from three sources: laboratory results, clinical expertise, and client preferences. These three sources are integrated to create an effective evidence-based practice.
- Without evidence or prior clinical experience, speech-language pathologists rely on working theories, trial-and-error, common sense, and their natural teaching ability to make clinical decisions about carryover.
- Most evidence on carryover actually concerns the topic of generalization. Virtually all of it reveals that each method works with certain clients.
- The little laboratory evidence we do have on carryover reveals that each method of carryover works for some clients some of the time.
- Generalization may be related to age and can occur from one language to another.
- Training a phoneme that contains a particular feature can stimulate production of another phoneme that also contains that feature.
- Both imitation and spontaneous speaking tasks can foster generalization.
- Phonemes can generalize to words when nonsense syllables are trained.
- A small number of words can be used to stimulate generalization of a phoneme to many words.
- Generalization can occur when parents and peers are involved in treatment.
- Generalization occurs equally when various syllable shapes are utilized.
- Generalization is promoted when clients have more general phonological knowledge.
- Self-monitoring techniques can facilitate situational generalization for carryover.
- Situational generalization can be facilitated with motor-based treatment approaches.
- Rapid production of word lists can facilitate generalization.
- Generalization can occur from one word position to another.
- Word-position generalization may not occur in clients with mental retardation.
- Word-position generalization may not occur in clients with severely restricted phonetic inventories.

Chapter 3

Managing the Carryover Process

"If the individual can engage in talking, and can think more of the subject than of the manner of his speaking, and yet have the manner correct, he has established control. Practice toward this end should be part of the training program and should be started as soon as possible."

– Mildred Berry and Jon Eisenson, 1956

This chapter begins our discussion of the methods and procedures of carryover. In this chapter we present broad ideas about managing the general process of carryover. We shall discuss balancing work and play, when to begin carryover, frequency of therapy, following the traditional plan of articulation therapy, functional work, speech contracts, parents, exercising patience, and many other practical ideas that work together in the management of the carryover process.

Balance

Carryover may be in jeopardy when work and play are not balanced in articulation therapy. Too much practice on words alone will not create an effective carryover routine. Likewise too much game playing will not assure the consistent performance needed for carryover. Speech-language pathologists balance work and play so that there is a natural give-and-take between rehearsal and relaxation, between practicing and playing, and between focused attention and distractions. Managing carryover means that some sessions are very drill-like and void of games, while other sessions are completely playful. Most sessions artfully combine the two. A balance of work and play is an excellent environment for stimulating carryover because it assures that the client is integrating practice and functional performance. Work and play are integrated to stimulate carryover.

Beginning Carryover Activities

When should carryover procedures begin? This is a controversial point and various beginning points have been suggested throughout the decades as a result:

- Some therapists have suggested that carryover begin after the client has mastered the new phoneme in words. For example: "When the child incorporates the sound into words easily, he is ready to begin the transfer to his everyday speech" (Eisenson and Ogilvie, 1965, p. 247).
- Some therapists have advocated that carryover begin once a client can say his new phoneme correctly. For example: "Carryover can begin as soon as the child has gained voluntary control of his sound and is able to produce it correctly at will" (Powers, 1971, p. 899).
- Some therapists have written that carryover should begin as soon as the client begins to self-monitor. For example: "When [a client] begins to listen to himself and hear that his production is different, carryover preparation has begun" (Bosley, 1981, p. 110).
- Some therapists have advocated that carryover procedures begin as soon as therapy starts. For example: "Actually the carryover process begins at the initiation of treatment" (Weiss, Gordon, and Lillywhite, 1987, p. 279).

My years of clinical experience have taught me that the last idea in this list is the best. It is my opinion that carryover should be built into the very fabric of a therapy program beginning with the first session. This view is based on my own three decades of practice.

For example, consider the client in therapy to remediate his deviant R phoneme. The first day of therapy may teach the client only one thing — that he is enrolled in therapy to learn to say R. To begin carryover immediately means that this first meager message must be carried into the broader aspects of his life. How? This is where the art of therapy comes into play. Perhaps the client will be guided to write an R in the middle of a paper, and then to draw a *rabbit*, a *robot*, and a *radio* around it. The page may be taken home and fastened to the refrigerator for the family to marvel over and for him to explain. The client naturally will say his R sounds incorrectly as he explains the picture to his family, but he will be connecting his speech work into his life. He will say, "This is what I am going to learn."

Cognition

Cognitive skill plays an important role in the carryover process. In fact, I have been known to say that low cognitive skill is our greatest deterrent to articulation improvement and carryover skill. As mentioned in our chapter on research studies, a few studies have demonstrated that children with lower cognitive skills do not generalize the way average children do. In the public schools in the 20th century, children were classified by cognitive level, and it was a commonly accepted notion that children who were below average did not generalize well. Generalization itself was considered the very skill that divided average learners from those that were below average. If it is still true that children on the lower end of the cognitive range do not generalize well, then we should expect that carryover would not be as successful with those children.

My experience has taught me that children with lower cognitive skills must be taught very specific skills under very specific circumstances. For example, take the situation of a seven-year-old student, who functions cognitively more like a two-year-old, and who is learning to produce B in words. This child may not generalize the B he learns on the word *bye-bye* to other words like *ball*, *baby*, or *big*. The child may have to be taught to say B on each word as it emerges individually.

In prior decades, speech-language pathologists turned to school psychologists for information about their clients' cognitive levels, but this information is not always available anymore. Today the SLP often must make his or her own general analysis of a client's cognitive level during the course of articulation treatment. I use the following areas to make a general determination of a client's cognitive status:

- Ability to follow directions
- Ability to answer questions
- Level of play skills
- Conversational speech skills
- Interests, likes, dislikes, and hobbies
- Receptive language testing scores
- Receptive reading level
- Any other formal test results that may be available

Contracts

It was popular in the 1970's for speech-language pathologists to make speech contracts with adolescents who were considered for articulation therapy. The client could attend treatment only if he signed a contract that he was willing to do the work all the way through to carryover. Teens made their own decisions about whether to continue therapy based on whether or not they were holding up their end of the contract. The thinking was that it does no good for a parent or therapist to make this decision for a teen or pre-teen. The child has to make this commitment himself. Contracts are an excellent addition to therapy when the carryover process is dragging.

Many therapists who submitted ideas for this book explained that they still use contracts today. In some situations, however, the old-fashioned speech contract seems to have been replaced by the Individualized Educational Plan (IEP). But the IEP is a contract with a parent and not a student. Speech contracts are made with the students themselves. A contract gives a client the opportunity to stay in therapy or to opt out. Some clients do quit, but simply knowing that quitting is an option is enough to keep many clients invested in the process. Clients who do not sign the contract, or who simply don't want to be there, are dismissed. No grudge is held in this regard. Clients are let go with the knowledge that they can change their minds at any time. They are told that the therapist will check in on them at a certain point to see if they are ready to begin the process. I have used contracts with children in both formal and informal ways. In many cases I simply ask, "Do you want to do this now?"

Controlling the Phonetic Environment

Traditional writers taught that we should control the phonetic environment of practice material in order to assure completion of an articulation therapy program. For example, consider S in the words *miss* and *mitts*. A client who can say one of these words correctly cannot necessarily say the other one correctly because the phonetic environments are different. Phoneme S occurs after T in *mitts*, but it occurs after a vowel in *miss*. Some clients cannot generalize speech motor skills this easily, and this makes carryover a problem. The traditional plan of articulation therapy is designed to usher our clients into carryover by carefully controlling the phonetic environment. For example, notice that only words that end in TS are used throughout the following increasingly difficult levels of treatment. Notice that the levels of therapy progress from simple to complex. Also note that there are no other target phonemes in these samples. The target is TS in the final position:

- WORD LEVEL: *Mitts*
- SIMPLE PHRASE LEVEL: *Two mitts*
- LONGER PHRASE LEVEL: *Two mitts and two hats*
- SIMPLE SENTENCE LEVEL: *Lenny got two green mitts.*
- LONGER SENTENCE LEVEL: *Lenny got two green mitts and two brown hats.*
- MORE COMPLEX SENTENCE LEVEL: *I think Lenny got two green mitts and two brown hats on Friday afternoon.*
- PARAGRAPH LEVEL: *My brother Lenny got mitts and hats on Friday afternoon. I went with him. It's the truth. Hats and mitts. He got both. He got green mitts and brown hats. I think he got two bats too! What's up with that? It's not fair. I thought he only could get the mitts, but mom let him get the mitts and the hats and the bats! I wanted new hats and mitts and bats too. That's only fair. Right?*
- STRUCTURED CONVERSATION LEVEL: Talk about one word from the paragraph above. Ignore all other S words as you talk.
- UNSTRUCTURED CONVERSATION LEVEL: Talk about anything. Ignore all S words that do not occur in the TS combination at the ends of words.

When therapists control the phonetic environment this tightly as in the traditional plan, we can take a client's production of his target from words to phrases, sentences, paragraphs, and conversation all within the same session. This is because we eliminate the need for generalization. We focus on one type of phonetic environment and we carry him through to conversation with it alone. This sweeps a client toward conversation very nicely quite early in therapy. Careful control of the phonetic environment is a very functional way to stimulate for carryover.

Frequency of Therapy

The frequency of therapy often plays into the carryover process. In general, most would agree that therapy that is spread out too thin is not good for speech learning and carryover. How frequently an individual client should attend therapy in order to promote carryover is a subject of considerable debate. Many today would argue that more frequent shorter therapy sessions are preferable, and this is a method that many old-timers advocated as well. The process of using more frequent and shorter sessions works well in the public school setting. But this idea is not practical in the private practice. For example, a private practitioner could not ask a parent to drive 45 minutes to and from therapy three days per week in order for their child to attend for five minutes each time. In general, clinicians must evaluate the ongoing needs of their individual clients and their unique therapy settings to determine how often therapy should take place for their clients to be successful in carryover. Periodic monitoring of carryover will allow one to measure whether therapy is taking place often enough for the individual client.

Functionality

It is generally agreed today that the more functional the articulation work is, the more assurance one has that new articulation skills will transfer outside of the therapy room. But there is a misconception today that old-time speech correctionists only worked on drill. This simply is not true. To read the old literature is to discover that speech-language pathologists have always understood the need to work functionally for carryover of newly learned speech skills. Consider these early admonitions to work functionally:

- *1912*: Scripture wrote one of America's earliest articulation therapy textbooks. The book contains three parts, and the entire third part is devoted to functional work, or what he called *exercises*. The text includes admonitions to work on speech using song, stories, talks, lectures, demonstrations, telephone calls, job interviews, store purchases, spelling activities, reading aloud, making introductions, and so forth (Scripture, 1912, p. 194-223).
- *1947*: Van Riper's earliest books also contain advice about working functionally. He wrote, "Practice of words in word lists will produce little transfer to real speech situations unless those words are taken out of their series and made part of the actual communicative function" (Van Riper, 1947, p. 207). "Motivation, maturation, discrimination, and application to life situations are indispensable adjuncts of any therapy" (Van Riper, 1954, p. 261).

As these quotes reveal, functional training always has been a part of our work. The old-timers taught that speech skills first are taught in a more isolated and structured environment, and then the work is taken into gradually more unstructured environments to promote carryover.

Unfortunately, beginning in the 1980's, some professional speech-language pathologists came to believe that articulation therapy only was valuable if it was perpetually tied to the narrative — "Articulation serves the overall process of verbal communication, and its rehearsal should always be related to communicative tasks" (Hoffman, Schuckers, and Daniloff, 1989, p. 256). Related to this was a new belief that the only way to make speech work functional was to work in the classroom. Astonishingly, some public schools today have gone so far as to ban speech-language pathologists from pulling children out of their classrooms to work on speech individually or in small groups because it is believed that training in a separate speech room is not functional. Traditional therapists disagreed with this notion. They believed that it was not the setting or the size of the group that makes our work functional — it is the process. Functional work can take place anywhere and with anyone.

If you have been caught in the *functional-therapy-can-only-take-place-in-the-classroom* routine, then step outside of the profession for a moment to think about how this idea might apply to another learning area. Consider the act of learning to tie shoelaces. Is it only functional if the child learns to tie his shoes when he's getting ready to go somewhere? Isn't it functional when a child goes alone into his bedroom to practice tying his shoes? And isn't it also functional if someone else comes into the room to give him a few pointers? I hope the reader can see that all these activities are functional for the child, they all serve their purpose, and they all carry the child toward complete functional use of the skill in everyday life.

Perhaps we could use the phrase *aspects of functionality* to refer to these divisions of functional learning. Articulation therapy entails various aspects of functionality that carry the client toward carryover. Our job is to make sure that what happens in the therapy room is valuable, and this occurs when articulation is learned through these aspects of functionality. Sometimes we drill on individual phonemes in isolation, and other times we work on syllables, words, phrases, sentences, reading, and conversation. Speech-language pathologists of the 21st century recognize that all levels of treatment are valuable for the client, and that it is the therapist's job to assure that all aspects of functionality are being addressed so that carryover can be achieved.

Parents, Caregivers, Teachers, and Aids

Parents, caregivers, teachers, and teacher aids can help in the carryover process, but it is a mistake to assume that they always can help. Having others involved may be the ideal, but parents and others vary in their parenting skills and teaching ability. We cannot expect all parents and significant others to be equally helpful in speech correction. The modern therapist understands that some of these people are helpful right away, some can be taught to be helpful over time, and others simply should be kept out of the process all together. Such is the nature of working with real people. Adjustments to the carryover process are made accordingly.

> *"The speech-language pathologist must first make a judgment about whether a parent will work positively with the client before embarking on a training program with the parent"* (Weiss, Gordon, and Lillywhite, 1987, p. 290).

It also is a mistake to assume that parents always need to be involved since some research has demonstrated that children often show equal progress at home and clinic. When parents can be involved in carryover, I like to give them simple and very concrete things to do during the course of everyday living. Parents are very busy people these days, and adding more homework to their evening routine often is impossible. I find that using key words works best. I also like to teach parents how to play with sounds and words with their children. Many ideas for involving parents are offered throughout this book especially in our last chapter on games and activities.

Bernthal and Bankson (2004) recommended that parents provide good auditory models, that they have their children practice words they already can pronounce correctly, and that they learn how to reinforce their child's correct productions. They also said that if parents are to be involved, they must be trained to judge accuracy of sound, they must be taught to carry out the procedures of the program, and they should be provided with written instructions. Hodson and Paden (1983) used parents to engage in auditory bombardment at home. The client plays quietly while a parent reads a word list containing the week's phonological target: "He only listens; he must not repeat the words" (Hodson and Paden, 1983, p. 66).

Peers / Speech Pals

Many therapists who submitted ideas for this book discussed ideas about using peers in therapy. The oldest reference we have for this seems to be a program called *Speech Pals* described by Erleen Marquardt (1959). Based on the theory that children learn better from their peers, and that other children are pace-setters, Marquardt's program had children of the same age or older assigned to speech students in the carryover phase. She gave suggestions about the type of students that make good Speech Pals. She said to select a child with good speech, and one who is bright, a natural leader, popular, and who can arrange their schedule to attend speech classes with their assigned speech student one time per week. Marquardt said, "It is necessary to make sure the Speech Pal has a disposition that will fit him for this type of helpfulness" (p. 156). Marquardt's Speech Pals were assigned to the speech student for the full school year. Their job was to attend class with the speech student one time per week, to learn about the speech process from the therapist during the session, and to listen to the speech student read out loud with good speech for a few minutes every day outside of therapy.

Modern speech-language pathologists continue to use modifications of the old Speech Pals program. Some of these pals today do actual teaching. Others simply serve as reminders to the speech student. Some Speech Pals use hand signals to cue their buddy to use correct speech in class.

Marquardt discussed several positive results of the Speech Pals program. She wrote that it benefits the client by attaching him to the popular crowd, and it benefits the Speech Pal who learns to use his or her natural teaching abilities. She also said that the program helps the school by desegregating the speech-impaired, it helps the community by bringing speech handicaps out into the open, and it assists special education in particular because it helps interpret the meaning of special education to the public. Marquardt said that her Speech Pals program was so popular, the therapists involved were met with this greeting every fall: "May I be a Speech Pal this year?" Speech Pals do not always have to be children with perfect speech of course. Fellow speech students can be used to help one another too.

Patience

A critical aspect of the carryover process is patience. We must remember that some of our clients are learning something that is very hard for them, and that it is easier for them to do it the old way. Charles Van Riper warned that we should not rush the carryover process:

> *"Most speech correctionists have to train themselves to resist this urge to hurry. When the child has been taught to make the new sound, the utmost patience and restraint are needed ... A lisper who has said 'yeth' for 'yes' several thousand times cannot be expected to say the latter as soon as he has learned to make the S sound in isolation"* (Van Riper, 1954, p. 248).

I remind myself of this need for patience by periodically engaging in a simply activity: I write my name with my non-dominant hand, and I make myself do this several times in one day. It's fun for a while, but then the drudgery sinks in. Do I have to do it like this? Can't I just do it my old way? The activity gets frustrating and even boring after a while, but it reminds me to be patient with my clients. It prompts me to give my clients time to mess up and time to get used to the process. It encourages me to slow down and let the carryover process continue at a pace of its own.

Review and Reflection

Many therapists stimulate carryover by reviewing work at the beginning and end of each session. Review and reflection is the process of talking about remediation and change. Review and reflection forces a client to think through what he has been learning and bring to mind the reasons he is attending therapy. These activities tie up loose ends and solidify the client's knowledge of the material. Review and reflection help the learner organize concepts and bring together the big picture for carryover. These are the conceptual exercises that teachers have done throughout time immemorial. The ability to think through one's work has been called *metacognitive skill* or *metacognitive knowledge*:

> *"Self-regulation for carryover is facilitated by students' development and the use of reflective thinking before, during, and after performances ... Without reflection, learners may fail to transfer metacognitive knowledge and strategies for improvement to new situations and tasks"* (Ertmer and Ertmer, 1998, p. 74).

Creating an old-fashioned speech binder that contains papers of the client's on-going work makes for an excellent speech review and reflection mechanism. This and other ideas for reflection are presented in our final chapter.

Measuring Success

How do we know when the carryover process has been successful? It has been recommended that carryover is complete only when the client can use his new speech skill in conversation both inside and outside of the therapy room. To measure success, Winitz (1975) recommended that carryover be assessed on a weekly or biweekly basis during 5-10 minutes of spontaneous speech both inside and outside of the therapy room. Therapists debate about the amount of success necessary to prove carryover has been achieved. The following three ideas have been prominent:

- EMERGING SKILL: The first view is that carryover will succeed when a new speech skill begins to emerge in spontaneous speech. In my experience, this measure can be sufficient only when very young children are first acquiring new phonemes. Once a typically developing small child begins to use a new phoneme spontaneously, carryover can be assumed in most cases. However this meager measure probably will be insufficient for older children with specific articulation deficits.
- PERCENTAGE CORRECT: The second view is that carryover is complete only when a client uses the new speech skill correctly to some predetermined percentage of correctness in conversation. No criterion has been established for this percentage, however, and it differs from one therapist to another. Should the criteria be 25%, 50%, or 75%? The word *consistently* has been employed to describe this: "The maintenance phase may be considered complete once the client can consistently use target behaviors in spontaneous speech" (Bernthal and Bankson, 2004, p. 286). I have always used 75-90% correct in spontaneous speech as my criteria of success.
- NEARLY 100% CORRECT: The third view is that carryover is complete only when a client uses his new speech skill correctly virtually all the time in conversation. Bosley wrote, "I was taught that the client was not through with speech training until he was carrying-over the new phonemes into conversational speech of all kinds nearly 100 percent of the time" (Bosley, 1981, p. 123). Most would agree that the goal of 100 percent of the

time is not measurable. Therefore we are talking about nearly 100% of the time in a sample of spontaneous speech.

*

Chapter 3 Summary

Managing the Carryover Process

- Carryover may be in jeopardy when work and play are not balanced in articulation therapy.
- Various points have been suggested for carryover to begin: phoneme, syllable, word, phrase, sentence, and conversation.
- The present author believes that stimulation of carryover should coincide with the beginning of therapy.
- Children with lower cognitive skills do not generalize well and carryover may not ensue. These children may need to be taught very specific speech skills under very specific circumstances.
- A speech contract gives a client the opportunity to opt out of therapy. Simply knowing that quitting is an option is enough to keep many clients invested in the process all the way through carryover.
- Therapists must evaluate the ongoing needs of individual clients to determine how often therapy should take place for carryover to be successful for each individual client.
- It has long been agreed that the more functional the articulation work is, the more assurance one has that carryover will succeed.
- Parents, caregivers, and peers can help in the carryover process, but it is a mistake to assume that they always can help.
- Sometimes the best way to manage the carryover process is to be patient.
- Many therapists review work at the beginning and end of each session in order to stimulate carryover.
- It has been recommended that carryover is complete only when the client can use his new speech skill in conversation both inside and outside of the therapy room.
- Therapists debate about the amount of success necessary to prove carryover has been achieved.

Chapter 4

Self-Monitoring for Carryover

"A consciousness of personal speech habits is mandatory in any improvement program."

– Johnnye Akin, 1958

A client's self-evaluation of his own performance is critical to carryover because this is the way new skills are monitored in all speaking situations. As we discovered in our first chapter, professional speech-language pathologists ranked self-monitoring as the most important aspect of a successful carryover program. Most of the activities in this book will help build self-monitoring of speech skills. However, this chapter focuses on ideas designed specifically for developing this skill. We discuss self-monitoring, auditory self-discrimination, conscious awareness, checking devices, correcting the therapist, daydreaming, exaggeration, and other methods.

Monitoring Oneself

Self-monitoring, or monitoring oneself, has been discussed widely in books on traditional articulation therapy, and is regularly mentioned as an essential component of carryover. Self-monitoring also been called *auditory self-monitoring* and *auditory self-evaluation*. Van Riper and Irwin called this the skill of *self-hearing* and *simultaneous auditory feedback*. They wrote, "[Clients] must learn to listen to themselves during the act of speaking" (Van Riper and Irwin, 1958, p. 127). Virtually all the writers of traditional articulation therapy in the mid-20th century discussed self-monitoring as a necessary and hugely important aspect of carryover. As noted in the first chapter, auditory self-monitoring was judged by speech-language pathologists in one study to be the most important element of successful carryover (Polson, 1980).

Auditory self-monitoring should be taught from early in therapy, but the process changes somewhat when we begin to use it solely for the purpose of stimulating carryover. We are referring here to the client who has full control over his new productions as long as he is thinking about them, but who fails miserably when he forgets about them. It is at this point of treatment that the client no longer needs to practice his phonemes. He must learn instead how to monitor himself consistently as he speaks in a wide variety of situations. He needs to learn how to recognize when communication partners are having difficulty understanding him, and how to take the time necessary to repair his errors during conversations.

Multisensory self-monitoring: The modern speech-language pathologist recognizes that self-monitoring is more than auditory. It is tactile and proprioceptive as well. A client's utterances have to feel correct as well as sound right. Self-monitoring is taught by studying the similarities and differences in the tactile, proprioceptive, and auditory realms of sound production. A multisensory focus should aid the carryover process. This basic therapeutic perspective has been understood for decades. Van Riper's work consistently included ideas about whispering, pantomiming, and wearing masking devices in order to encourage attention to proprioceptive feedback.

> *"The most important automatic controls for monitoring articulation are proprioceptive. These controls see to it that we use the right movements, the right postures, the correct contacts"* (Van Riper and Erickson, 1996, p. 250).

Auditory Self-Discrimination

A critical component of self-monitoring is auditory discrimination of one's own correct and incorrect productions, a process sometimes called *auditory self-discrimination*. Discrimination of one's own speech is different from, and usually more difficult than, discriminating someone else's speech. This is what can make carryover difficult to acquire. Therapists usually begin by teaching a client to discriminate the therapist's productions. Then they teach the client to discriminate his own.

> *"It is not enough for the case to be able to recognize the correct and incorrect speech sounds as they are spoken by other people. We must also help our cases to hear themselves, to listen to their own mouths"* (Van Riper and Irwin, 1958, p. 116 and 123).

Auditory self-discrimination is encouraged by asking clients to judge their own performances. We ask: How did you do on that one? Do you think that one was correct or incorrect? Did you forget on that one, or did you remember? Did you do that one the way we have been practicing? Questions like these transfer the decision-making process from us to them. This is the very skill our clients need for carryover outside of our therapy rooms. Encourage the client to listen to himself by saying something like, "I want you to listen to yourself. Let's do it again. Listen to yourself very carefully because I am going to ask you if you did it right or wrong."

Conscious Awareness

Self-monitoring of speech for carryover also involves a conscious awareness of what is going on in therapy. Does the client understand why he is coming to speech? Does he realize that he is coming to learn something, or does he think that it is just for games? Most traditional writers suggested that conscious awareness is a key to carryover.

> *"The student must know what he is trying to do throughout the whole therapy"* (Van Riper, 1947, p. 207).

> *"In order to change his speaking patterns, the client must become keenly aware of the areas of speech to be changed ... The trouble spot must be made to stand out dramatically"* (Bosley, 1981, p. 110 and 113).

There is no one single way to help clients come to this awareness of their speech goals. Instead there are lots of ways to go about it depending upon the client's age, cognitive level, interests, and other factors.

School-age students can be asked certain questions to stimulate conscious awareness. For example, ask, "Why did you come here today?" It does no good if a client answers, "Because it is 10:30," or "Because the teacher said it was my turn," or "Because I want to play the robot game again." The client must be able to explain the real reason for attending speech, and his answer must be specific. He needs to say he is coming to speech "to fix my R" or "to practice my S." A specific answer like that allows us to know that the client really understands the process. I ask my clients a question like this in just about every session, and I help them formulate a correct answer. When a client starts getting a little upset because the question is being asked too often, then I know that he really understands what we are doing and I begin to back off.

A different approach will be needed to develop conscious awareness of the purpose of therapy in very young children, in those with low cognitive skills, and in any other clients who cannot answer a question about why they come to speech. Most clinicians rely on simple statements, boisterous praise, and mutual imitation to give these clients an idea of what's going on. Consider the following dialogue in Table 1 (on the next page) as a demonstration of this with a client who is functioning at approximately 18-months of age. Read the dialogue line-by-line from left-to-right as the conversation unfolds. Cues about the techniques being employed are found in the right-hand column. Simple dialogues such as this bring clients with limited levels of speech and language performance to a conscious awareness of the purpose of therapy.

Checking Devices

Van Riper wrote about the use of *checking devices* for building self-awareness of speech productions (Van Riper, 1947, p. 203). Checking devices are used by clients to record the number of errors they make during a certain time or activity. For example, Van Riper suggested that a client carry an index card and pen. Every time he notices that he has made an error he marks a tally on his card. Another interesting suggestion Van Riper made was for the client to keep marbles in a pocket. Every time he makes an error the client transfers a marble to the other pocket. This becomes a simple way to count his errors. Records are kept for the number of errors the client makes, and he is rewarded for making fewer as time progresses. A mechanical or electronic clicker counter or tally counter could be used today instead of marbles. A simple checking device can be a powerful tool for increasing awareness of habits outside of the therapy room.

I have used a checking device in my own process of speech therapy. I was diagnosed with a vocal cyst in 2009 after having neglected the health of my own voice throughout many years of public speaking. I began voice therapy on myself, and then enlisted the help of another pro-

Table 1 – The "Bye-Bye Dialogue"

Child With A Cognitive Level Of 18 Months	Therapist	Techniques
Bye-bye.	Bye-bye. Yeah! (With clapping)	Mutual Imitation Positive reinforcement
Bye-bye.	Bye-bye! Good job.	Mutual Imitation Positive reinforcement
(silence)	Bye-bye!	Model
(silence)	Bye-bye... You do it.	Model Demand for performance
Bye-bye.	Bye-bye! Kristina said *bye-bye*.	Mutual Imitation Building a concept of what is going on in therapy.
(silence)	You are learning how to say *bye-bye*.	Building a concept of what is going on in therapy.
Bye-bye.	Bye-bye!	Mutual Imitation

fessional SLP. One of the first things I recognized was that the irritation of the cyst had caused me to develop a habit of clearing my throat many times per hour, especially when teaching. Throat clearing and other habits were causing my folds to swell, and aphonia often was the result after a day of teaching. I began treatment on myself by tallying the number of times I cleared my throat during certain periods of the day. I could not believe it when I discovered that I was clearing my throat upwards of 30 times in a 15-minute period! That meant that I was banging my vocal folds together at least once every thirty seconds! Tallying my throat clearings shed light on this aspect of the aphonia. When I began therapy with the other therapist, she suggested that I train myself to swallow instead using the hard glottal attack. One month later, I used the checking device again, and this time found that I had reduced the number of throat clearings to only 4 times in 15 minutes. This was a significant improvement. The checking devise had had an immediate positive effect on my self-awareness of the problem. This allowed the substitute pattern to be incorporated almost immediately.

Auditory Events

Sounds in the environment can be an effective way to stimulate self-monitoring during the carryover process. The hearing of the sound causes the client to think about his speech. Engel et al (1966) called these signals *auditory events*. Auditory events might include a telephone ringing, a school bell chiming, the sound of a car whizzing by, the child's name being called, someone saying "Hi," or a dog barking. Select one environmental sound and help the client become aware of it. Try to select one that will occur often. For example, a school chime is an excellent reminder in the upper grades because of all the class changes. The client uses the auditory event to remind himself to use his good speech.

Daydreaming

Some clients do not monitor their own speech for carryover because they do not understand how good speech fits into their future. Helping a client think through his own personal dreams and aspirations can be a powerful tool in the process of building self-awareness and carryover. Daydreams are a tool we use to carry our lives into the future. Therapists can use daydreaming as a way to help clients build their conscious awareness of their future with good speech.

I am reminded here of a young boy, nine years of age, who did not want to attend speech classes for his distorted R. He intended to become a professional basketball player and play for the Chicago Bulls, and he did not see how correcting this error fit into his dream. This boy was little and scrawny, and probably had very little chance of ever becoming a professional basketball player, but instead of squashing this dream, I fit the speech work into it.

One day I said to him, "Man, wouldn't it be cool if you actually could play for the Bulls? Excellent. You might win the NBA playoffs! … What if you won the playoffs, and you were the star player on the team? … That would be amazing! And what if the reporters all wanted to interview you after the game? ……… You wouldn't mind talking in front of millions and millions of people with that incorrect R?"

The boy thought for a moment. I could see in his eyes that he was imagining the moment when the championship game was over and he was the victor. In his mind he was holding the trophy in his arms and the reporters were approaching him for their interviews. After a moment of imagined revelry, the boy changed his mind and said, "Okay. Let's do it!" He worked hard all the way through to the process of carryover. I am sure this boy's daydreams about winning the championship carried him along even though the topic never was brought up again.

Fitting articulation therapy into existing daydreams can be a solid way to ensure carryover, therefore therapy has to be unstructured enough that therapists can figure out what their client's dreams are. If the new speech production fits into the client's dreams about his own life, then he will work toward carryover without much more help from us. But he may balk until it does. We have no laboratory evidence to prove this, of course. Using a child's hopes and aspirations is a classic teaching method that we can apply to the carryover process.

Demonstrations

Children can come to greater self-awareness of their own speech when they demonstrate their newly learned skills to others. A demonstration is a display, show, or performance of skill. I have found this to be a most effective carryover procedure. Each skill the client learns, no matter how simple, can be demonstrated for someone else besides the treating therapist. Helping a client gain confidence in his new skill by showing off to someone else takes away the notion that new speech skills are to be kept secret. Demonstrations can be put on all the way through therapy, from beginning to end.

There are countless ways to demonstrate skills depending upon clinical setting. Our clients can demonstrate to other children in their group. They can demonstrate for siblings or parents invited into the room, or at home. They can perform in front of their teachers or other adults in the school or clinic. They can perform in front of a small group or a large class. They can show off their skills to dolls, toy soldiers, or stuffed animals lined up on a couch. They can perform for puppets we wear on our hands. They can perform while making video or audio recordings to be shown at home or posted on the Internet. Mirrors can be used to practice demonstrations or to substitute for the presence of other people.

Distractions

Periodic distractions during therapy routines can be effective in stimulating self-monitoring for carryover. Speech-language pathologists purposefully distract a client while he is in the middle of speaking correctly. This knocks him off track so that he is at greater risk of making an error. The client is given cues or hints as necessary to help him recover. For example, we might interrupt the client's productions with a series of boisterous (fake) sneezes. Distractions like this are not intended to knock the client off track permanently. Distractions are intended to teach the client how to stay on track despite them, and they are intended to knock the client off track so he can practice getting back on. This idea was born of the present author's clinical experiences.

Exaggerating the Error

A client's exaggeration of his own error also is an especially good procedure to engage the process of self-monitoring for carryover. Have the client produce his error louder, longer, quieter, with bigger movements, or with greater pitch and intonation variations. This method can be fun, but it also must be done with sensitivity. We do not want the client to get the impression that we are making fun of him. This is a technique that has been recommended time and again in books on traditional articulation therapy: "Through exaggeration, conscious awareness of both the articulatory activity and acoustic product is created" (Berry and Eisenson, 1956, p. 161).

Hardest Words in the World

Some clients do not work toward the end of therapy because they cannot visualize that there will be an end. Speech-language pathologists have to help clients build a concept that there will be an end to therapy, and that the end involves speaking any and all words with their target sound correctly. This can seem like a very big and un-attainable goal to a child, therefore we need a way to make the end more concrete for him. I do this by helping my clients create a list of words that we call *The Hardest Words in the World.* I use this list to help the client visualize the end of therapy and the carryover it will entail. The words on this list are the difficult ones that the client encounters on a regular basis.

Most children come to therapy with at least one word that is driving them crazy because it is very important and they cannot say it correctly. Perhaps this troublesome word is their own name, or the name of their favorite sport or after school activity. Perhaps this word is the name of a book they must report on next week, or it is a word in a passage they have to recite in front of the class. Perhaps this important word is their age that they cannot pronounce well when people persistently ask, "How old are you?"

We can start building the list of the hardest words in the world with the one or two words the client is concerned about at the onset of therapy. I usually ask, "Are there any words that you cannot say and that are really bugging you?" We add new words to the list as treatment progresses. I teach my clients that therapy is just about over once they can say these words freely and easily with anyone with whom they talk. This gives the client the end goal, and it teaches him that that end goal is accomplished outside of the therapy room.

The hardest words list is a powerful motivator I developed throughout more than three decades of service. I have found that many clients take every new skill they learn in therapy and apply it immediately to their list of hardest words. This process of leaping forward to skills for which they are not quite ready is quite helpful for connecting the present work to the client's life. The process is helpful even if the client fails, because if he fails, he will return the next week and ask how to do it. I have found that determined clients will try to use whatever skill they have learned to figure out these troublesome words, and they practice persistently until they figure it out. Then, as soon as the client succeeds, he transfers the new production immediately into the conversations in his life that require it. Practicing a client's own personal set of hardest words is one of the most powerful motivations for carryover I have ever found. The hardest words list drives the client forward because he no longer wants to be embarrassed by his lack of skill on these specific words. It drives him into and through the carryover phase with almost no additional prodding.

Imitating the Error

A very effective method of forcing a client to examine his own productions is to imitate his error. This technique is discussed in many classic textbooks on articulation therapy, including Van Riper. It is a technique my professors taught me, and one I continue to use to this very day. The process goes like this:

- Model the client's error: "You are saying it like this…."
- Then model the correct production: "Most people say it like this…."

The method is an effective one for clients who have no clue that they are saying a sound incorrectly. It also is good for clients who know something is wrong but they can't put their finger on it. Some clients respond with shock when they hear the way they really sound, but imitating the client's error is not intended to shame or embarrass them. Our purpose in imitating a client's error simply is to awaken him to it. Imitating a client's error must be done with discrimination and sensitivity. It is not done in front of other children, and it is employed in ways that do not interfere with rapport.

The process of modeling a client's incorrect production takes a certain level of skill on the part of the SLP. The client's error must be imitated exactly for it to be of real value. Therapists get better at this with time and practice. Imitation of the client's error can be a real boon to self-monitoring in the carryover process when we can do it correctly. Audio or video recording the client's error is another way to accomplish this.

Information

Information about the need for carryover helps build the client's self-monitoring skills. A client may come to therapy twice per week and practice hundreds of words that contain his target sound, but this alone may not help him understand that he is supposed to say the sounds correctly anywhere else. We must tell him. This is a process of bringing the problem of carryover out into the open by describing it instead of correcting it. For example, in teaching L we might say, "You have to say the L sound correctly when you speak with everyone."

Valerie Frost-McKinley has an interesting way of giving information to her clients about the need for carryover. She tells them that their words have to paint a clear picture for their listeners. She tells them that if words are not spoken clearly, or sounds are misarticulated, then the listener receives a fuzzy picture or message. With this idea firmly established, she then teaches parents and teachers a prearranged sign or words to let the student know when they haven't received a clear picture. Explicit information about the necessity of carryover helps children develop the concept of carryover itself. Information helps the client learn what his responsibility is in this regard. This is a common sense teaching idea that has had broad application in all fields. We give our clients information about what is expected of them so they can make a choice about change.

> *"When grownups describe the problem, it gives children the chance to tell themselves what to do... Information is a lot easier to take than accusation"* (Faber and Mazlish, 1980, p. 57-58).

Key Words and Phrases

Once a child can produce a correct sound in words, it is natural to expect him to say it correctly all the time in his everyday speech, and some parents, teachers, and therapists begin to nag children to use their new correct sound all the time. Van Riper said that they should not nag but "concentrate their reminding and correcting upon a few common words" (1954, p. 258). Today we call these words *key words*. Bosley (1981) called them a *core vocabulary*. Marti Fuller and Philip Shively were among many professional speech-language pathologists who contributed this idea to our website. Marti uses the term *magic words*, and Philip calls them *anchor words*. Key words, core vocabulary, magic words, or anchor words are words that occur frequently and have high functional value to the client. They are words that we expect the client to speak consistently correctly outside of the therapy room.

For example, when working on final S, the word *please* is an excellent choice for a key word. It is a word that a client has opportunity to use many times per day. It also is a word that the client can *make* opportunity to use many times per day. Key words can be practiced in therapy, and then plans can be made for using them correctly outside of therapy. This is a fantastic production activity that many therapists use the world over. Start with one or two key words, and build the number in the set over time. Put your head together with the client and his family to identify functional words that contain target phonemes and are the most frequently occurring in their home. Write the word on an index card and send it home to fasten to the refrigerator. Teach the parent how to elicit that word at least once per day every day. Key words might be divided into basic sets as follows:

Words With Highest Value

Key words and phrases that children need to use all the time:

- PERSONAL INFORMATION: The child's name, age, and grade.
- PEOPLE AND PETS CLOSE TO THE CHILD: The names of people with whom the client interacts the most including parents, siblings, and other people living in the home, as well as pets and close friends.
- IMPORTANT ADULTS WITH WHOM THE CLIENT HAS REGULAR CONTACT: Teachers, coaches, sitters, other relatives, neighbors, and activity leaders.
- ADDITIONAL PERSONAL WORDS: E-mail address, telephone number, address, and birthday.

School Related Words

Key words that are important for school functioning:

- SUBJECTS: The names of classes he takes as well as the names of the other periods of the school day.
- COMPUTER: Words and phrases related to computer use for school work are very important today — *software, hardware, save, copy, paste, program, Excel, Word, Apple, PC, spread sheet, boot, re-boot, sign on, sign off, look up, search...*
- ALPHABET: The names of the alphabet letters.
- NUMBERS: The numeral names, including the hundreds, thousands, and so forth. Also words for math functions.
- CLASSMATES NAMES
- PRINCIPAL, OTHER TEACHERS, AND STAFF NAMES AS NEEDED

Words With Broad Communicative Value

Key words that have very high functional value are those that are sprinkled throughout just about any dialogue or conversation:

- GREETINGS: Words and phrases of greeting — *Hi, Hey, Bye, See ya, See ya later, Catch ya later...*
- COMMON SOCIALLY COURTEOUS WORDS: Pleasantries we use to be nice to others — *Please, Pretty please, Thanks, Thanks a lot, Thank you, Thank you very much, Excuse me, May I...*
- POSITIVES: Words and phrases that are used to agree — *Yea, Yes, Yep, Okay, Sure, Uh-huh, I do, Wow! Nice! Excellent! Cool! Man! Yes! All right! I think so...*
- NEGATIVES: Words and phrases that are used to negate — *No, Nope, No way, Uh-uh, Never, Not, I don't, I don't know, I don't think so, Are you kidding! Forget it, Sick! Yuck! Terrible! Gross! Disgusting!*

- NON-COMMITTALS: Words and phrases that do not commit to an idea — *Oh, Uh-huh, Hmm, I guess, Whatever, Maybe, Could be, I don't know...*
- CLARIFICATIONS: Words and phrases that are used to get more information — *Wait, Hold on, What? Say what? What's that? Huh? Really? What did you say? Say that again...*

Household Chores, Routines, And Furnishings

Words that are of very high value at home are those that involve household routines, meal preparation, chores, homework, bedtime, and so forth. For example, if the target phoneme is F, we might chose functional phrases like *Feed the dog, Turn it off, Channel five, Fried chicken, French fries, In the 'fridge, In the freezer, Found it, Finished it*, and *Fix it.*

Semantic and Syntactic Forms

Words and phrases that also are of very high value in the carryover process are those grammatical forms that occur regularly, especially:

- PRONOUNS: Words that stand for people (and animals) about whom we talk — *I, me, my, mine, you, your, yours, he, him, his, she, her, hers, we, our, ours, they, them, theirs...*
- COPULAR AND AUXILIARY FORMS OF TO BE: Word forms of the verb of existence and action — *is, am, are, was, were, be, isn't, aren't, wasn't, weren't...*
- QUESTION WORDS: Words used to ask questions — *who, what, where, when, why, how, how come, how many...*
- CONJUNCTIONS: Words and phrases that join two ideas together — *and, but, because, so, so that, then, and then, before, after, as soon as...*

Extracurricular Words

Key words that identify or are related to broader aspects of the child's life.

- SPORTS: Words that name and describe the client's sports activities, positions, and players — *basketball, swimming, soccer, baseball, tennis, first base, kick, throw, touchdown, quarterback, coach, hoop, dunk, jump shot, assist...*
- COMPUTER: Words related to computers for extracurricular activities are very important today—*on-line, off-line, e-mail, Twitter, Facebook, YouTube, Internet, website, blog...*
- GAMES: Words that name the board games, word games, computer games, and neighborhood games that the client plays at home with family and friends — *jump rope, Monopoly, X-Box, hangman, tag...*
- ENTERTAINMENT: Words that name the clients favorite television programs, movies, cartoon figures, and actors — *Superman, Batman, Sesame Street, Elmo, Mickey Mouse, SpongeBob SquarePants...*
- INTEREST GROUPS: Words that name and describe the people and events of social interest groups — *scouting, camping, choir, badges, ceremony, meeting, fund raising, event planning...*
- BIRTHDAYS: Words about birthdays — *present, party, cake, candles, games, friends...*
- RELIGION: Words and phrases of the client's religion — *Sunday school, confirmation,*

high holidays, bar mitzvah, Passover, Christmas, Ramadan...

- HOLIDAYS: Words and phrases — *Fourth of July, Independence Day, Martin Luther King, Jr. Day, Presidents' Day, Memorial Day, Labor Day, New Year's Day...*
- VACATIONS: Words for upcoming times off — *camp, camping, tent, hotel, pool, horseback riding, grandma's house, Disney World, Six Flags...*

Nucleus Situations

Van Riper had another substitution for parental nagging to promote self-awareness and carryover. That is to employ a *nucleus situation* (Van Riper, 1947, p. 204). This means to correct the child only when he is in a certain place or setting at home. For example:

- Correct the child only when he is sitting in a certain chair.
- Select only one person with whom the client has to use his new speech skills every time he talks with him or her.
- Select a certain specific situation during which the client must speak correctly. For example, require the client to use his new speech skills during dinner or while riding in the car.

Van Riper suggested that these nucleus experiences would cause the child's new skills to spread rapidly to all other situations. He suggested that when errors occur in one of these nucleus situations, the child should be penalized vividly but in a friendly way. Correcting a child only during certain nucleus situations can be difficult for some parents. They may feel like they are doing nothing when they are not correcting. Help parents get past this by asking them to think about the way their child learns other things like spelling, math, or soccer. Help them realize that the child will burn out and tune out if he has to do any of these things all day long. Ask them to think about how they felt when their own parents rode them about certain chores or activities. Help them learn to back off. Teach them that there is a time for math, a time for spelling, a time for speech correction, and a time to ignore these things.

Preparatory Mindset

Bosley suggested that the process of carryover is assisted when children are trained in a *preparatory mindset* (Bosley, 1981, p. 122). For example, she suggested setting a rule about good speech like this: "As soon as you leave my room, you are to speak correctly, using your new sound." Bosley suggested that such a rule would build a self-awareness of expressive speech behavior. Rule setting is especially effective with children who are very rule-bound.

I am reminded of one young client who had four interrelated problems: A persistent and very severe habit of thumb sucking, a persistent infantile suckle-swallow pattern, an anterior open bite, and multiple misarticulation errors including a frontal lisp. At his three-year checkups, both the pediatrician and the dentist said that his thumb sucking was not a problem. This bright and very literal boy took them at their word. He took his thumb out of his mouth when I was working with him in therapy, but he would not comply with the idea of quitting thumb sucking all together because the doctors said it was okay. The next year, however, at his four-year checkups, both the doctor and the dentist did an about-face, and said he needed to quit the thumb sucking. The boy completely quit the next day. Rule-bound children like this can adapt nicely to many new ideas when people they trust explain pertinent rules in terms they can understand. This is a standard teaching method that we can apply to the carryover process.

Questioning Progress

I have found that posing questions to clients about their progress is an effective tool to stimulate self-awareness for carryover. Example questions might include: How are you doing on this? Are you figuring this out? How is this speech work going for you? Are you thinking about this work when you are at home… at school… in band practice… while out with your friends? Question like these force clients to think about their speech in broader contexts. Many children answer "I don't know" to these questions and they need to be encouraged to think harder. If they cannot answer, tell them straight out, "Oh, you have not been thinking about this. I want you to think about your speech. Use your brain. Get those brain cells working!" Help them figure out the answers to these questions. This puts their mind on the carryover issue. This is an old-fashioned, tried-and-true teaching method. In my school days our teachers said, "Put on your thinking caps!"

Prodding

Many speech-language pathologists prod their clients during therapy conversations to promote self-awareness of speech for carryover. To prod is to nudge, hint, poke, incite, encourage, or remind a client to use his correct speech productions while he is in the act of speaking. This is an untested method of stimulating carryover into conversation. It is used at just the right time during conversation. Prodding can be multisensory. Consider the following examples of prodding that might be used with a client who has been working on S. The client can say the sound correctly, but he needs to be prodded to remember to say it the right way as he is telling his therapist about a painting he has completed:

- VERBAL PRODDING: The therapist says the letter S periodically as the client tells her about his painting.
- VISUAL PRODDING: The therapist pantomimes production of S as the child talks about his painting.
- AUDITORY PRODDING: The therapist audibly says the sound of S periodically as the child describes his painting.
- TACTILE PRODDING: The therapist gently touches the client's chin periodically as he talks about his painting.
- WRITTEN PRODDING: The therapist writes a reminder letter, word, or symbol on an index card and places it on the tabletop. She points to the card periodically as the child explains his painting.

Recordings

We can use audio, video, and computer recordings to promote both auditory and visual self-awareness. In the 1950's, therapists began to use tape recorders to provide *delayed auditory feedback* to build auditory self-monitoring skills: "The delayed scrutiny of samples of his own speech can aid greatly in activating his self-hearing" (Van Riper and Irwin, 1958, p. 127). Recordings provide several advantages as described so well by Van Riper and Irwin:

> *"The mere act of recording his speech helps the case get set to listen, makes him pay some attention to the speech itself, and permits him to hear it again and again ... The delay helps the case to be objective, to assume an experimental attitude in his scrutiny. Errors and correct sounds may be experienced again and again ... Most cases, as they listen to their own speech, tend to follow it empathetically, by moving their lips and uttering the words silently. This tendency can be used to good advantage"* (Van Riper and Irwin, 1958, p. 126).

Reminders

Self-awareness for carryover can be enhanced when reminders are used. A reminder is a visual cue that the client uses to jog his own memory regarding correct speech. The old-fashioned idea of tying a string around one's finger is an example, and more appear below. This is a standard psychological method used to break old habits or to establish new ones. Clients can design these themselves, or we can help them determine the best reminders. The beauty of a visual reminder is that the client himself may be the only one to know what the reminder means.

One client developed a reminder system that no one in his family ever realized was a reminder. Steven wrote himself a reminder on a sticky note that said, "Steven is cool!" He placed it on the home computer. He told his family that he just wanted to remind them how cool he was every time they went on-line. But then his brothers wanted to say something positive about themselves too, so they replicated the note using their own names. The idea became a family practice. Family members were hiding positive notes about themselves all over the house in places like coat pockets and cookie jars. Each found note became a further reminder for the client to use his correct sound at home, yet no one in the family knew that this was the first note's original purpose. The following reminders also can be a secret:

- CARTOON CHARACTERS: Select one cartoon character the client likes as his reminder about carryover. This is a great idea for little kids who are attracted to cartoon characters. For example, perhaps the child adores SpongeBob SquarePants. The SpongeBob depicted on his pillowcase, lunch box, notebook, or jacket becomes a reminder to use his new sound.
- DOTS ON PAPER: Teach an older client to draw a tiny dot in the middle of each paper he is working on. The dot is unobtrusive and not recognizable to anyone else. Teach the client to draw the dot first thing each time he starts a new paper. The dot reminds him about his new speech sound.
- DOTS ON HANDS: Teach a client to draw a tiny dot in a visible place on his hands. The client draws the dot first thing in the morning, when first sitting down at the desk in school, when beginning homework, and so forth.
- BAND-AIDS: A band-aid worn on a finger can be a nice unobtrusive reminder. Make sure to change the location of the band-aid every day to prevent extended dampness on that part of the finger.
- STICKERS ON THE SCHOOL BINDER: Place a sticker on the child's 3-ring school binder as a reminder. Place additional stickers on each tabbed divider of the binder so he will see

them when he flips through from section to section.

- STICKERS ON TEACHERS AND PARENTS: Contributor Ricki Block has teachers and parents wear reminder stickers on their shirts. The child sees the reminder every time they interact. Some teachers and therapists wear aprons. Stickers and pins can be worn there too.
- BRACELETS: Bracelets can be used as reminders. Yoela Holman uses paper bracelets she buys at an office supply store. The bracelets have a few lines where the therapist or student can write a reminder message. Being made of paper, these bracelets are worn for as long as possible. One also might use a silicone support bracelet for longer use. The bracelet itself may be enough, or use a permanent marker to write the target letter on it.
- STICKERS ON CELL PHONES: Linda Richardson reminds us that older children can place sticker or dot reminders on their cell phones. With the way young people are glued to their cell phones these days, this may be the best modern-day carryover idea yet.
- TEMPORARY TATTOOS: Tattoos are a controversial subject, but temporary tattoos are popular among children and can be used to remind them of their speech work if you are so inclined. Obtain parent permission first and drop the idea if it seems objectionable to the client himself. Chose an appropriate image, for example, a robot for R.
- NOTES AROUND THE HOUSE: Have the client place a sticky note or an index card reminder in places around the house. Place one on his desk, his computer, on his headboard, or on the bathroom mirror. The note can say anything, really, as long as the client knows that it is a reminder to use his new sound.
- PHONETIC PLACEMENT CARDS: Tamara Seeker has children make cards with instructions about phonetic placement for use as reminders. The children write out their instructions in their own words. For example, a client who has learned to say R might write, "I need to walk my tongue tip back along the roof of my mouth, tighten, and say my good R." Then three copies of the cards are glued to three index cards and laminated. One is for home, one for their desk in the classroom, and one is for the teacher.
- POWER CARDS: Denise Prohaska submitted the idea of using Power Cards for articulation carryover. The idea originally comes from a practical book about autism and Asperger syndrome (Gagnon, 2001), and Denise adapted the idea to articulation carryover. The idea is to use an index card on which the therapist and client draw a picture of a character or person in whom the client is interested. For example, the client might draw Superman. Then a few sentences are written about how that individual uses good speech. Then three "I statements" are written about how the client will use his speech sounds correctly. The card is laminated and placed on the client's desk. The student starts his day by reading the card. The card acts as a reminder throughout the day. Teachers and aides can reference the card periodically to remind the client to use his new speech sounds.
- SOFT POUCHES: Jennifer Code gives her clients a soft crocheted pouch that they wear under their clothing as a reminder about their speech.
- SHAKE UP THE WARDROBE: Donna Ridley has kids alter their wardrobe or hair to help them remember their speech work. For example, the child might wear only one sock, or wear the hair up instead of down, or wear jewelry that is not usually worn, or not wear jewelry that usually is, or wear a watch on the opposite wrist.

- CLOWN FACES: Chana Hartman makes laminated clown faces as reminders in the student's classroom. The clowns have large mouths, oversized hats, a bow tie, and two hands. Lamination allows her to write on the clowns with erasable markers. She writes successful target words on the hat, new words still being practiced on the mouth, and notes about special hand cues on the hands. The clown is hung in the classroom where the child and others can see it. She says the clowns help her keep teachers informed about what is going on in speech. Other images could be used as well.
- OTHER STUDENTS: Several therapists who responded to our call for ideas wrote that they used other students as reminders. Every time they see that student they remember to use their speech correctly.
- THERAPIST PICTURE: Many speech students switch to better speech as soon as they see their speech teacher. As a result, many therapists use pictures of themselves posted in the classroom as reminders. The picture can be posted to a bulletin board or to a client's desk.
- FACIAL EXPRESSIONS: Teach the client to read facial expressions and body language so they become reminders about his speech.

Self-Cues

An excellent way to build a client's self-evaluation skills is to develop a cue he will use to remind himself to use his new speech skill outside of the therapy room. Cues can be formal ones found in published programs, or they can be self-designed. I actually prefer that my clients make up their own cues because these will be the most meaningful for them.

An example of a successful cueing system used in carryover comes from my own experience. I was working on slowing rate of speech with one teenage boy who could speak intelligibly as long as he remembered to slow down. He was controlling his rate by tapping a pencil eraser on our tabletop to mark each syllable of the words in his conversations. I asked the client to do this in class and elsewhere, but he wanted a cue that was less obvious. He said he would prefer to tap his finger on his leg, or in his pocket. What an excellent idea! The client had devised his own cue to help himself control rate outside the therapy room. After a few weeks, the client asked if he had to keep using the finger-tapping method. When asked why, he complained, "I can do it in my head. I don't need to tap my finger any more." Excellent. The pencil-tapping cue, and then the finger-tapping cue, helped him carryover his control of rate just as they were intended.

Simultaneous Tasks

Van Riper suggested the use of what he called *simultaneous tasks* to promote self-monitoring for carryover. The idea is to work on speech and do other simple activities at the same time. This is done to teach the client how to keep his mind on his speech while otherwise engaged. For example, Van Riper advocated that clients talk while writing or drawing (Van Riper, 1947, p. 201). I have used this method all throughout my career and have found it to be an excellent method for carryover in clients of all ages. Little children especially like to draw while talking, and boys in particular seem to participate better during speech tasks when then have something in their hands with which to fiddle. Gross motor activities done in conjunction with speech work always have been recommended as a stimulator of carryover. For example, have the kids hop, jump, skip, hula-hoop, bounce a ball, or bounce on a large ball while practicing speech words.

Speech Assignments / Scripts

Van Riper recommended what he called *speech assignments* to promote self-awareness for carryover. Speech assignments are simple tasks assigned to the client during which he will use his new speech production skills purposefully outside of the therapy room. For example, Van Riper suggested having the client go to another adult in the building and ask for an object whose name includes the target word. He also recommended having the client say a target word three times to another child during another part of the day without the other child knowing that he is doing it, or having the client ask his parent if he said a word correctly: "The teacher should always make these assignments very definite a[illegible]opriate to the child's ability and environment" (Van Riper, 1947, p. 203).

The speech assignment often i[illegible]ipt is a written draft of the words that will be spoken between the cl[illegible] short, planned dialogue. Scripts are written together with the [illegible] *who, what, where, when, why,* and *how* of the assignment.

- WHO: To whom will he [illegible]
- WHAT: What will he say [illegible]gue?
- WHERE: Where will this lit[illegible]ue occur?
- WHEN: When will this little [illegible]logue occur?
- WHY: What is the reason for speaking to this person?
- HOW: How will the dialogue track if the client speaks correctly? Incorrectly?

Therapists must make sure that clients return the following session with news about how their speech assignment went. If a client forgets, try to get him back on track with a little prodding. Help the client determine a cue to help him remember to carry out his speech assignment. Ventures into the rest of the world on speech assignments can be scary for some clients. Therefore it is important to identify safe people with whom to have these dialogues. The concept of the safe person is discussed more in our chapter on personality, emotion, and attitude.

Client Input

A powerful means to develop a client's self-awareness of his need for carryover is to encourage him to develop his own method. Ask the client, "How are you going to remember to do this when you are not with me?" Most clients have some notion about how they remind themselves about chores, homework, and other activities. Perhaps they keep a calendar, put a note on the refrigerator, or set an alarm. The idea here is to encourage the client to design his own plan for carryover. This is not a way for a therapist to be lazy about designing a plan. It is simply that a client may know best how this idea will fit into his own life style.

It should be noted that a client's own ideas were judged by therapists to be one of the least effective means of carryover (Polson, 1980). It is hard for me to understand why this would be except that perhaps it was not common practice for therapists to solicit client ideas at that time.

*

Chapter 4 Summary

Self-Monitoring for Carryover

- Self-monitoring has been discussed widely in books on traditional articulation therapy, and is regularly mentioned as a necessary component of carryover.
- Therapists have judged self-monitoring as the most important aspect of carryover.
- Self-monitoring is auditory, tactile, and proprioceptive.
- Posing questions to clients about their performances can be an effective tool to stimulate auditory self-monitoring for carryover.
- Most traditional writers advocated that conscious awareness is a key to carryover.
- Checking devices are used by clients to record the number of errors they make during a certain time or activity.
- Auditory discrimination of correct and incorrect productions has long been considered a critical component of self-monitoring and carryover.
- Helping a client gain confidence in his new skill by showing off to someone else builds self-monitoring and takes away the notion that the things learned in the speech room are to be kept secret.
- Self-awareness of speech can be built when grownups describe the problem to the child. Information is a lot easier to take than accusation.
- Distractions are intended to teach a client how to keep his speech on track despite them. Distractions also are intended to knock a client's speech off track so he can practice getting back on.
- A client's exaggeration of his own error is an especially good procedure to engage the process of self-monitoring for carryover.
- A list of the client's hardest words helps him build an awareness of the end of the therapy process.
- Imitation of a client's error is an especially good way to bring it to his conscious awareness. Do this with sensitivity.
- Daydreaming can be used as a way to build a client's conscious awareness of a future with good speech. The client becomes better at monitoring himself as he envisions his future.
- Help clients self-monitor by encouraging them to concentrate on a few key words.

- Help clients self-monitor by encouraging them to concentrate on their speech during a few specific nucleus situations.
- Rules build self-awareness of expressive speech behavior. They are especially effective in the carryover process with children who are very rule-bound.
- Audio, video, and computer recordings can be used to promote auditory and visual self-awareness.
- Cues can be developed to help a client remember to use his new speech skill outside of the therapy room.
- Speech assignments, or scripts, are simple dialogue tasks assigned to the client during which he will use his new speech production skills outside of the therapy room.
- Asking the client to design and select his own methods of carryover can stimulate self-awareness.

Chapter 5

Speech Production Activities for Carryover

"Somehow we must build in this person a control system that will continuously scan the utterance and notice and correct the errors automatically."

– Charles Van Riper and Robert Erickson, 1996

A significant part of facilitating carryover has to do with the way speech is practiced during therapy sessions in activities we shall call *speech production activities*. A wide variety of speech production activities have been suggested for the promotion of carryover. This chapter discusses a number of them including babbling, chanting, disagreements, error play, fill-in-the-blank activities, negative practice, nonsense material, and so forth. These ideas come from traditional books on articulation therapy, my own clinical experiences, and from ideas submitted by practicing therapists. Ideas are presented in alphabetical order with no hierarchy implied. They can be used in therapy or at home.

Babbling

Babbling is perhaps one of the most widely used production activities in articulation therapy. Van Riper used the term *strengthening* to refer to the carryover process, and he suggested that we use babbling to insure this strengthening: "One of the most effective methods for strengthening a new sound is to include it in babbling" (Van Riper, 1954, p. 249). Van Riper was not advocating babbling as a method of stimulating new phonemes in young children, the way most of us use it today. He was suggesting that we use babbling as a method of carryover in high-functioning articulation cases. Van Riper suggested that babbling should be used this way once a client has gained his new phoneme. He said that this type of babbling should contain a wide variety of phonemes, and it should be free flowing and as effortless as possible. He stated that the target sound should not stand out within these babbling sequences, and that there should be no pausing before or after the sound. Van Riper was trying to get us to understand that babbling can help in the carryover process if the performed motor sequences are like the style of conversation — rhythmic, smooth, natural, quick and easy. He suggested that these sequences should not be tightly structured, but that the babbling should go where it will.

There was a period in our history when it was taught that babbling had nothing to do with mature speech. In fact, this was the prevalent view when I was an undergraduate student. But this notion was dismissed once we began to look more carefully at infant vocalizations, and when Oller (1978) stated that there seemed to be a direct relationship between the structure of babbling and that of early words. Since then most speech-language pathologists have used babbling regularly as a method of phoneme stimulation and stabilization.

The beauty of babbling is that it can be used to practice speech sequences that have no meaning other than the meaning of the sound sequence itself. A client can focus on the motor patterns of the babbling sequences without getting tangled up in the motor memories he has for familiar words. Babbling is pure motor speech practice. Babbling is not the end product, of course, and one cannot expect babbling to be the answer to all the client's problems with carryover. But babbling can be a means to the end.

> *"Since articulation is, in part, a motor process, having the client produce the correct sound rapidly over a number of trials may help the pattern to become more automatic"* (Johnson, 1980, p. 188).

Chanting

Chanting is a standard teaching method that has been used the world over since the beginning of recorded time. Chanting encourages carryover because it is mesmerizing. In my experience, chanting aids awareness, memory, retrieval, automaticity, and habituation of new material. Chanting is different than singing. To chant is to recite a word or phrase rhythmically and with a simple intonation pattern. Chanting creates a rhythm to speech movement that sinks deeply into the soul. Chanting frequently is done in unison by groups of people, and the reader may be familiar with religious chanting that is practiced in a quiet meditative attitude. But chanting can be done in a more child-like and boisterous way: "Words and phrases can be incorporated into chants to be used when walking or during calisthenics" (Bosley, 1981, p. 111).

Very verbal toddlers speak in a chanting way as they play alone and talk to themselves. For example, I heard one two-year-old who was playing alone with a doll chant to herself for about 40 minutes by saying: "My baby… My baby… My baby… My baby eats… Oh-oh baby… Oh-oh baby… Don't cry, baby… Don't cry, baby… Don't cry, baby…" Chanting solidifies a child's early speech and language foundations. Chanting can be a way to drill speech units in a rhythmic way while engaging in another activity.

Correcting the Therapist

An excellent way to help a client build self-awareness of his own productions is to have him correct the therapist. Say words purposefully wrong to pique the client's auditory attention. Act confused when he tries to correct you. Ask him to explain what the problem is. This forces him to become super aware of what you are doing wrong, and what you are doing right, and he will say the two sounds back-and-forth himself to discover the differences. This method also puts the client in charge for a change. "No one likes to be on the receiving end of correction all the time" (Bosley, 1981, p. 114).

Describing

Old-timers often recommended that clients be asked to say things about objects or pictures as a way to begin the process of spontaneous productions. For example, Scripture (1912) recommended that we place an object on the table and have the client:

- Name a word associated with the object. For example, the client might say, "Read," if the object is a book.
- Make a melodious statement about the object.
- Name the object and then another object in the room.
- Describe the object in a single word or in a sentence.

Many therapists who responded to our survey of ideas for carryover submitted ideas about using objects and pictures for clients to describe, so apparently this activity is still widely used today. Therapist suggested that clients could describe hidden objects, imaginary objects, objects they spy out a window, clothing, foods, toys, people, occupations, teachers, things on the playground, things in the cafeteria, movies, television programs, and so forth.

Disagreements

Scripture (1912) suggested that clients be taught to argue for stimulation of carryover. He suggested that we teach clients to remain cool while arguing with the instructor, with somebody else, in a group of three people, in a debate forum before a small group, and in a political debate.

Error Play

Playing with an error sound or word can be an excellent production activity and your ticket to carryover because it is so much fun. Just think about the joy a child experiences when an adult makes a funny sound or says a funny word! For example, once a child learns that a *sink* is called a "sink" and not a "think," it becomes fun to play with these differences. The child's father can joke around with him at home by insisting that there is a "think" in the bathroom. Or they can argue playfully about whether there is a "think," a "sink," or a "stink" in the bathroom. This is outstanding carryover work because it captures the child's attention and encourages entertaining practice away from the therapy room.

Playing with errors encourages auditory attention, awareness, discrimination, and memory. Playing with an error can be much more meaningful to the child than sitting down at a table to do the begrudged speech homework. Playing with error sounds or words is quick and easy, and it can be practiced a little bit here and there throughout the day. This also is a valuable skill to teach parents if they do not already interact with their children in playful ways. Playing with errors is functional articulation therapy at its best. Learning through play is a standard teaching method. In this case, we are showing the client how to play with phonemes and words.

Idioms

Idioms make a wonderful topic of discussion in therapy for the stimulation of spontaneous speech. An idiom is a fixed, distinctive, and usually colorful expression whose meaning cannot be determined from an analysis of its individual words. For example, consider the following expression: *It's raining cats and dogs*. This is an expression about how hard it is raining, not an expression about animals falling from the sky. Children usually love to learn about, talk about, and draw pictures that depict idioms. Books of idioms can be purchased, and many examples of idioms can be found on the Internet. Talk about what the idioms mean, where they come from, and how they evolved over time if known. Idioms stem from many languages in many cultures over many centuries, so they fit nicely into many classroom topics. A book of idioms is an excellent addition to any speech therapy room.

Model Self-Correction

Along with modeling a client's error comes modeling the self-correction process. Make a purposeful error and then make a big deal about fixing it. This draws the client's attention to the process of noticing one's own error, of stopping to think about it, and then of correcting it. For example, say, "Oops. I think I said that wrong. I said 'wady'. I should have said 'lady'. Let me try that again..."

Negative Practice

Van Riper discussed the use of *negative practice* as a speech production activity in the carryover process. Van Riper defined negative practice as "the deliberate and voluntary use of the incorrect speech sound or speech error" (Van Riper, 1954, p. 258). Sometimes the best way to break a habit is to do more of it for a certain time, and this is what we are doing with negative practice. Van Riper said that voluntary negative practice increases the client's vigilance in self-monitoring, and it acts as its own penalty because it becomes distasteful. He wrote that negative practice builds conscious awareness of the error: "Consciousness of the [error] must come before it can be eliminated" (Van Riper, 1947, p. 205). Van Riper's rules for using negative practice included:

- Help the client understand why you are using negative practice.
- Never use negative practice until the client has good mastery over the correct production.
- Imitate the client's error exactly when you engage in negative practice.
- Confine all negative practice to the speech session [i.e., do not use negative practice in the classroom in front of peers.]
- The client should learn to do this by imitating his error immediately after he makes it.
- Use the negative practice to serve the purpose of teaching correct versus incorrect productions.
- Use negative practice at all traditional levels: Isolated sounds, syllables, words, phrases, sentences, paragraphs, and conversation.
- Use negative practice to build auditory discrimination.

An entire session purposefully making target phonemes in error can be quite beneficial because children love it. Negative practice aids carryover because it causes the child to listen for the error in himself and others, it gives him the freedom to make the error after having learned the correct way, and it encourages conscious practice of the error and its correction outside of the therapy room. This is a very practical idea that has never been formally studied.

Nonsense Material

Many authors have recommended practicing nonsense syllables and words to strengthen the carryover process, and nonsense material has been shown to generalize to real words. Like babbling, nonsense words do not have auditory and motor memories attached to them, and "nonsense syllables pose less interference with previously learned behaviors than do words" (Bernthal and Bankson, 2004, p. 285). Nonsense material can do much to promote carryover because children think it is fun, because they often rehearse it outside of the therapy room, and because they usually want to share these ideas with family and friends. For example, use toys and make up names for them that exemplify the client's target phoneme. For example, to introduce stridency, use toys named *Sue*, *Shep*, and *Cho*. Use whatever type of toys the child likes such as stuffed animals, dolls, plastic dinosaurs, or puppets. Include these characters as participants in all other speech activities to encourage spontaneous production of the sounds. Babbling also can be considered the practice of nonsense material, and there are more ideas in our final chapter on games and activities.

Overpractice

To overpractice is to practice to excess, or to practice beyond the point of correction. Overpractice can be an effective production activity for carryover because it causes a hyper-awareness of the goals of therapy. Overpractice has been shown to be somewhat effective as a method of carryover (Bankson and Byrne, 1972).

I am reminded of a speech-language pathologist I met in Indiana who uses overpractice as a general therapy method. She makes her students pay their way into her speech room by rehearsing their sounds 100 times. She keeps a chart of the numbers on the wall next to the door of her therapy room. The children point to the numbers 1-100 as they say their sounds or words. This therapist told me that she originally designed the activity out of desperation because her caseload was so large and she saw the children in big groups. She needed a way to get enough data on each child every week, so she came up with the idea of the chart. At first she thought the kids would hate the idea, but she discovered that they loved it! The kids challenge each other to go faster and faster through the chart. If they make a mistake, they have to return to the beginning and start again. Imagine the hyper-awareness these students experience each week as they overpractice their speech by using the number chart. Once the children have paid their way in to the therapy room, treatment focuses on games and other activities that entail more relaxed conversational work.

Rapid-Fire Questions and Answers

Many therapists have suggested the use of rapid-fire questions and answers to stimulate practice for carryover. Ask questions to which there are single-word answers that contain the client's target phoneme. Ask the questions fast, and make the clients answer fast. Children usually love this type of interaction as it excites them. With increased excitement comes less attention to the particulars of speech production. Build speed and encourage clients to maintain correct productions for as long as possible until complete breakdown occurs at some point. After a good laugh, slow down and start over. This type of activity teaches clients how to hold their speech together while speaking faster. They usually love the challenge. Basic math practice is an excellent way to encourage rapid-fire questions and answers. For example, when working on prevocalic F:

- 3 + 2 = ___. (Answer: *5*)
- 60 – 5 = ___. (Answer: *55*)
- 20 – 6 = ___. (Answer: *14*)
- 101 + 3 = ___. (Answer: *104*)
- 500 x 3 = ___. (Answer: *1500*)

Reading Aloud

As we mentioned in our first chapter, reading out loud can be an excellent step along the way toward effective carryover, but it never should be considered the final product of a carryover program. This is because spontaneous speech and reading aloud are different in several ways:

- Reading is performed much more slowly than conversational speech. Reading aloud rarely matches the rate of conversation.
- Reading aloud involves orthographic symbols. These symbols function as cues for production.
- The process of reading out loud gives clients more opportunity to think about *how* they are speaking because they do not need to focus on *what* to say.
- Reading usually is less passionate than spontaneous speech.
- Reading someone else's ideas is not creative in the way that spontaneous speech is.

Reading aloud seems to act as a step between word productions and conversational speech. Reading to promote carryover is a common sense solution that can be found in some of our earliest texts. For example, one hundred years ago, Scripture (1912) suggested that reading activities should include poems, prose, dramas, sentences, statements, questions, and paragraphs. Have the clients read storybooks, classroom materials, or things they write themselves. Many therapists have clients highlight target words to help them focus while reading. They do this either by using pencil marks that can be erased afterwards, or by photocopying the pages and using highlighters and other colorful markers to make the words stand out.

Rapid Reading

Rapid reading has been suggested as a production activity to promote carryover, and rapid reading has been shown to transfer to conversational skills to varying degrees. Reading paragraphs can work well, but it is easier for children to speak increasingly fast if practice material contains rote syntactic structures. Use counting, the alphabet, word lists, simple song lyrics, or simple poems. Repeating phrase and sentence structures are my favorite way to encourage rapid reading. For example, when working on S:

- REPEATING PHRASES: A big spoon, a big sock, a big slide, a big snake…
- REPEATING SENTENCE STRUCTURES: I have a new spoon, I have a new sock, I have a new slide, I have a new snake…

Pretend Reading

Many clients cannot read in the true sense, but they can pretend to read by making up a story line to go with a book. This is a common technique for working with preschool children and other pre-readers or non-readers. Pretending to read might be considered a step between actual reading and spontaneous speech because the client is making up the words as he goes along. Many therapists like to use wordless picture books for this activity.

Reading Pictures

Children love sentences written with pictures that substitute for words. For example, the sentence *I see the sun* would have a picture of a sun in place of the word *sun*. Children love thinking through these word pictures. Make the pictured words be the target words. Sentences with pictures are a nice way to stimulate pre-reading in preschool children.

Fill-in-the-Blanks

Many therapists have used fill-in-the-blank sentences or stories as a way to stimulate reading for carryover. Gerber (1973) said that they can be used at all levels of therapy. Determine a single sentence to use throughout the entire activity. For example, pretend to fill a grocery bag with foods that contain the target sound. Have the client say, "I am buying a ___ and a ___ and a ___…"

Key Words Reading Activity

Use key words and have clients make up sentences in which words are missing. Write the incomplete sentences on cards and share them in the group for others to solve. For example, when working on L in all positions: "Lucky Lucy was riding her horse when she ___ off. Poor Lucy! She had to go to the ____ because she bonked her head. It seems that ___ wasn't ___ after all!" (Key words: *fell, hospital, Lucy, lucky*)

Rhyming Couplets

Recitation of simple rhymes has long been recommended as means of encouraging carryover. Working on rhymes can capture a client's attention, but the real beauty of a rhyme is that the client may memorize and practice it outside of therapy. Rhymes make a nice bridge from single words to conversation. Simple two-line couplets are nice to use, for example: "My teacher likes to teach; She teaches at the beach." Children can memorize two-line couplets easily, and they are motivated to share amusing ones with other children. Couplets that children write themselves are usually the most memorable. For example, when working on R, one client wrote: "Don't you dare fart; Down at the K-Mart." I am sure he practiced this couplet every single day and taught it to many other children outside of therapy.

Riddles

Riddles have been used the world over to teach children any number of new vocabulary words and ideas, and they can be used to stimulate carryover of new speech skills. A riddle is a puzzle in the form of a question or rhyme that contains clues to its answer. In the case of articulation therapy, the answer contains the target phoneme being stimulated. Riddles are an excellent method of carryover because they cause a client to combine practice material with creative thinking. Gerber (1973) contains a number of rhyming riddles designed specifically for carryover. Here are a few directly from her text as examples:

- For initial S: "Shiny and yellow and hot and bright. We see it by day but not by night." (Answer: *Sun*)
- For medial R: "It flies through the air. It's long and narrow. It's shot from a bow and is called an ______." (Answer: *Arrow*)
- For final L: "Throw me down, and up I go. I am rounder than an O." (Answer: Ball)
- For initial Sh: "It's like a big spoon attached to a pole. You use it when you want to make a hole." (Answer: *Shovel*)
- For medial Ch: "I have a handle and a spout. Tip me over and the water pours out." (Answer: *Pitcher*)
- For final Th: "I am part of your face, and here's what I do. I sing and I whistle, I talk and I chew." (Answer: *Mouth*)

Shortening Prolongations

Many speech-language pathologists have their clients prolong phonemes during practice in the therapy room. This helps clients attend to new phonemes, and to figure out how to produce them. The problem comes however when our clients always prolong new sounds during speech practice. Van Riper cautioned that prolonged sounds never carry over to conversation: "A sound which the student takes too long to produce will never become habitual" (Van Riper, 1954, p. 249). He suggested that we should encourage our clients to shorten their productions once they can produce them. Van Riper said that shorter productions should carry over more easily.

Singing

Songs have been used to educate young children the world over since the beginning of recorded time. Most 20th century articulation therapy texts recommended using songs to teach or to reinforce articulation skills when working with very young children or those with cognitive deficit. In a delightful book called *Sing Your Way to Better Speech* (1939), Gertrude Walsh published an entire articulation program in song. She quoted George Elliot: "Men's muscles move better when their souls are making merry music" (p. 1). I believe that the quote refers to hard labor produced by grown men, but the theory could apply to all people under all circumstances, including our speech clients who are working on carryover. Singing is useful for many reasons. Singing helps children remember sounds and words, it encourages children to practice almost without realizing that they are doing so, it is easy, it is an excellent way to work with children in groups or in the classroom, it easily carries over to other situations, and it is fun!

Change the Words

Walsh's model for using songs is a good one. Take a familiar tune and write new lyrics that contain words with the target phoneme. For example, to the tune of *Twinkle, Twinkle, Little Star*, one could emphasize initial P by singing:

Pinky, Pinky, Little Pooch.
Pretty puppy, give a smooch.

Put you paw right on my lap.
Please don't chew on my new cap.

Pinky, Pinky, Little Pooch.
Pretty puppy, give a smooch.

Use the Words

Songs also can be used with their existing words. Almost any song can be used for any purpose, however Karen Dickson offers the following old-time song-phoneme match-ups for later-developing phonemes and clusters. I have added a few additional phonemes to her list:

- *The Farmer In The Dell* — F, L, R
- *Mary Had A Little Lamb* — R, L, M
- *She'll Be Coming Around The Mountain* — Sh, K, R
- *Oh, Suzanna!* — S, Z
- *Skip To My Lou* — S, Sk, K
- *I've Been Working On The Railroad* — R, S, B, W
- *The Wheels On The Bus* — W, B, S, R
- *Head, Shoulders, Knees, And Toes* — H, Sh, N, T, Z
- *The Hokey Pokey* —H, P, R, L
- *Jack And Jill* — J, L
- *Old Macdonald Had A Farm* — O, M, D, F, M, E, I, O, and animal sounds
- *Five Little Speckled Frogs* — F, L, Sp, F, R, L
- *The Itsy Bitsy Spider* — S, T, B, Sp
- *Who Stole The Cookie From The Cookie Jar* — K, J, R
- *It's Raining, It's Pouring* — R, P, Sn, Ng
- *Five Little Monkeys* — F, L, J, K
- *Twinkle, Twinkle, Little Star* — Tw, L, St, R

Speed Up

Rate of production may be one of the most important variables during speech practice for the carryover process. Most therapists try to get their clients to slow speech down for the purpose of establishing carryover, and most writers in traditional articulation therapy recommend the same. We tend to think that a client could carry over his new speech skills if he just spoke more slowly out there in the real world. But telling a client to slow down usually doesn't work because clients will slow down for a few seconds and then speed right up again.

Hilda Fisher taught the opposite. Fisher was co-author of the *Fisher-Logemann Test of Articulation Competence* (1971) and she wrote a very popular textbook called *Improving Voice and Articulation* (Fisher, 1966). I heard Fisher speak at a conference on articulation and voice therapy when I was a very young clinician (circa 1978), and she said that slowing our clients down is only the first step. The second and more important step is to speed them up. She said we must make sure to build speed into the treatment plan because a client always will want to speak as fast as his peers. She said that speed is what induces carryover. Fisher taught that we should design games and activities that encourage clients to speak faster so they go beyond the point of breakdown. She said not to be afraid of breakdown, and not to avoid it. Instead, she said we should use games that tend to get faster and faster, for example, the card game called *War*. Structure the work so that the energy builds as the game continues. Teach the client to notice what the breakdown feels and sounds like as speed increases. Then teach him how to hold himself back from that point as the energy builds. In other words, the client's articulation naturally will deteriorate when he speeds up, so when it does, teach him how to notice it and how to pull back to a slightly slower rate so that he can avoid breakdown.

Fisher also said that we should teach the client to recognize his own personal speed limit. Challenge the client in this by telling him that you are going to make him talk so fast that he will make an error on every target. The client will try to prove to you that he can control his speech better than that. This is just like teenagers who need to drive too fast periodically in order to learn how to control a car's speed. Our clients need to speed up, make errors, listen to the error, understand the error, and then learn to control rate in order to avoid the error. The analogy to driving helps them understand this. As an additional note, Bosley advised that adjustments to rate of speech production often have to be dramatic for children to understand what we are talking about: "At first you may have to speed up dramatically before the child even notices" (Bosley, 1981, p. 113).

Spelling

Spelling can be used to encourage carryover from the beginning of articulation remediation. Practicing speech while spelling can be done in the therapy room, in the classroom, and at home. Spelling homework sometimes is the only time parents carve out time to work directly with their kids, so combining spelling and speech work is advantageous for carryover at home.

In therapy, spell out target words correctly while practicing them, and spell words incorrectly to reflect the way the client says them. Use these correct and incorrect spellings to discuss correct and incorrect productions. For example, when talking about *soup*, say, "You said, *thoup*. Watch… T… H… O… U… P… Is that what you meant? Or did you mean *soup*? S… O… U… P… Which one did you mean to say?" Spelling out errors is an excellent way to help the client stop to think about what he is saying and how he is saying it. Spelling is a way to integrate articulation work and literacy. Spelling is an untested method has been used to promote articulation and carryover since Van Riper. He had kids spell words and pronounce the sounds at the same time: "The most important of all strengthening devices is the use of simultaneous talking and writing. In this procedure, the student writes the script symbol as he pronounces the sound" (Van Riper, 1947, p. 197).

Story Telling and Re-telling

Many speech-language pathologists use story telling and re-telling to stimulate carryover skills. Story telling and re-telling function like steps between reading aloud and spontaneous speaking. These activities allow the client to take a small step away from reading. Children can tell and re-tell the stories of any published children's novel. Picture books without pre-written story lines can be used to have clients create a story. Children also can be encouraged to draw pictures as they make up their own stories. Focus on the speech production and the story plot together. Story telling is a common teaching method that can be employed in the carryover process. Story telling has been discussed in some of our earliest texts: "Read aloud a short story … then with the book open before you, relate the contents of the story" (Scripture, 1912, p. 220).

Error Stories

What often makes story telling and re-telling really fun is allowing kids to do a loose re-telling so that the facts get confused. This is fun in a group. Let the kids make up parts that were not in the original story, let the other children jump in to correct the story or to add incorrect facts, or let the whole re-telling be completely wrong. Add more fun by having the kids tell an opposite story, or have them tell a story backwards. Children love this creative process. It encourages them to hold their speech together while ideas become increasingly imaginative.

Story Maps

Lisa Anderson has her clients make story maps for creating stories in the carryover process. A story map is developed by writing down one word, and then writing down as many other words or phrases the kids can think of that relate to that first word. The first word should be one of the client's target words. For example, the target word might be *robot*. Around that word might be *metal, computers, automatic, man-made, Star Wars, R2D2, C3PO, space ships, aliens, planets, space travel, science, independent, cool, The Terminator, I want one*, and so forth. Once the map is made, it is used to generate sentences, paragraphs, or a story with the target word as the central theme. The stories then are treated as any other reading material.

Story People / Stick People

An excellent way to help young children tell familiar stories for carryover is to make *Story People on Sticks*. Take a picture book and photocopy pictures of the main characters. Color them (or make color copies), cut them out, laminate them, and staple them to tongue depressors to make people on sticks. Now you have each character of the story represented as a stick puppet. The stick people are manipulated as the kids tell the story. Provide doll furniture and other accoutrements for more help and more fun. The story people on sticks can be kept in the speech room for special times, or the children can make them as an art project to take home for carryover story telling with their families. Send the stick people home with a list of the main words, or with a copy of the story itself with highlighted target words. For example, make a Momma Bear, Papa Bear, Baby Bear, and Goldilocks stick figures. Then use 3 doll bowls, 3 doll chairs, and 3 doll beds as props. Children love this.

I started doing this years ago when I had a client who would talk about nothing but *The Wizard of Oz*. After trying dozens of ways to get him to talk freely, I finally gave up and bought a book that had photographs from the movie and made my stick people. The client was thrilled and jabbered away each time we used them.

Story Starters

Karen Dickson uses stories starters for helping children write stories from scratch for stimulation of carryover. These ideas come from *The Reading Teacher's Book of Lists* (Fry, Polk, and Fountoukidis, 1984) and other sources:

- I looked around the room. Nothing seemed unusual, but then ...
- I never expected that one day I'd open my closet and find ...
- It was three times as large as me, but I was going to try anyway ...
- I never thought I could do it, but ...
- This couldn't be the truth because ...
- If time could stand still, or even go backwards, I would ...
- It was an ugly animal but I loved it because...
- It was Christmas morning, but I was not anxious to ...
- My dog jumped up and started barking ...
- It was my best friend's deepest secret and it would be a hard one to keep ...

True/False Story Game

Mollie Marlow has her kids play a story-telling game for carryover. The game requires that each child hold two cards. One card has *True* written on it and the other has *False*. To play, one child tells a story, and that story can be a true story or it can be a lie. The child telling the story selects his *True* or *False* card, and places it face down on the table. This is his mark of the type of story he is telling. As the other students listen, they decide whether they think the story being told is true or false. The listeners select the appropriate true or false card to place face down on the table, too. When the story is finished, the therapist turns over all the cards to see if any match. Each student who guessed correctly whether the story was the truth or a lie gets a point for that round. The game continues for a certain length of time or until one player reaches a certain number of points. More than one winner can occur in each round. The therapist and students judge each other's speech throughout the game.

Tongue Twisters

Children like to use tongue twisters to learn how to control their speech. We have no research on the effectiveness of these sayings, but tongue twisters are fun, they pique auditory self-monitoring, and they seem to be a nice bridge between reading and spontaneous speech. A wide variety of tongue twisters can be found in children's books, children's workbooks, or on the Internet. Consider creating your own by using the phonemes and phonological patterns you are teaching. Have children say the target twister one time, or have them repeat it many times in sequence. Work on increasing speed in order to twist the tongue up nice and tight. For example, I modified these from tongue twisters I found on-line:

- FOR INITIAL K: "Can you can a can of clams as quickly as a canner can can a can of clams?"
- FOR INITIAL R: "Robert Ronald Robin robbed Robyn Ronald Robert. "
- FOR INITIAL KL BLENDS: "Clean clams were crammed in clean cans."
- FOR S IN ALL POSITIONS: "Six sick hicks nick six slick bricks with six slick sticks."
- FOR INITIAL W OR FINAL SH: "I wish to wish the wish you wish, but if you wish the wish the witch wishes, I won't wish the wish you wish to wish."

*

Chapter 5 Summary

Speech Production Activities for Carryover

- A significant part of facilitating carryover has to do with the way speech is practiced, rehearsed, or drilled during therapy sessions. We have called these speech production activities.
- Association games are an excellent way to stimulate spontaneous production of words, phrases, and sentences.
- One of the most effective methods for strengthening a new sound is to include it in babbling.
- Chanting seems to help with awareness, memory, retrieval, automaticity, and habituation for carryover.
- Playing with an error sound or word can be an excellent production activity for carryover because it piques auditory discrimination and is so much fun.
- Sometimes the best way to break a habit is to do more of it for a certain time. This is called negative practice.
- Many authors have recommended practicing nonsense syllables and words to strengthen the carryover process because nonsense material is not associated with prior learning.
- Overpractice can be an effective production activity for carryover because it causes a hyper-awareness of the goals of therapy.
- Many therapists have suggested the use of rapid-fire questions and answers to stimulate carryover.
- Reading out loud can be an excellent step along the way toward effective carryover, but reading aloud never should be considered the final product of a carryover program.
- Rapid reading has been suggested as a production activity to promote carryover.
- Recitation of simple rhymes has long been recommended as means of encouraging carryover.
- Riddles have been used the world over to teach children any number of new vocabulary words and ideas, and they can be used to stimulate carryover of new speech skills.
- Van Riper suggested that shorter productions should carryover more easily than prolonged productions.
- Most 20th century articulation therapy texts recommended songs to teach phonemes and to stimulate carryover.

- Increasing speed of speech production induces carryover.
- Spelling is a way to integrate articulation and literacy for carryover.
- Many speech-language pathologists use story telling and re-telling, with and without errors, to stimulate carryover skills.
- Children like to use tongue twisters to learn how to control their speech.

Chapter 6

The Role of Behavior Modification in Carryover

> *"A newly acquired sound ... is usually rather unstable. One minute the case can utter it perfectly, the next minute it is gone."*
>
> – Charles Van Riper and John Irwin, 1958

Carryover is possible only when clients are engaged in a consistent behavior modification program. Behavior management is based upon positive and negative feedback given to the client in response to his performances. As we discovered in our first chapter, professional speech-language pathologists ranked consistent behavior management as the third most important aspect of a successful carryover program. In this chapter we shall discuss basic concepts of behavior management as they apply to carryover.

Identify the Goal

Behaviors that are identified are easier to change than behaviors that remain hidden or unnamed. This means that speech-language pathologists must have a clear goal in mind, and this idea must be transmitted to the client: "The client must identify the habit to be broken" (Bosley, 1981, p. 109). Identify and set a specific goal, write it out in the client's paperwork, and help him iterate it. Try to establish a clear goal for the client during the evaluation process or very early in therapy. Create a visual representation of the client's goal. For example, have the child write his target sound (letter) on the whiteboard next to his name. Teach clients that they are attending therapy in order to learn to say their target sounds correctly all the time. This is a fundamental concept of behavior management that most writers of traditional articulation therapy said had an important role in the carryover process.

Practice, Rehearsal, and Drill

There has been much naysaying about the negative aspects of drill in articulation therapy, but practice is used the world over in any process of skill habituation and behavioral change.

Pianists use practice to habituate key-striking skills, dancers use rehearsal to habituate leaping and turning skills, and basketball players use drill to habituate ball-handling skills. Practice, rehearsal, and drill are very important aspects of skilled movement habituation. Speech also is movement. Therefore, most therapists have viewed practice, drill, and rehearsal as important methods of speech habituation. Many therapists hope that practice, rehearsal, and drill in the therapy room will be all that is necessary to induce spontaneous carryover of new speech sounds. It certainly is nearly all that is needed when we work with easy clients.

Virtually all the old-time articulation textbooks recommended practice, rehearsal, or drill. In fact, some very early writers insisted that *persistent drill* was necessary to assure carryover: "Before discharging the patient the instructor should … fix the results of the treatment by persistent drill on selected exercises [in order to] develop the patient's tentative and uncertain production of the new sound into a firmly rooted speech habit" (Borden and Busse, 1925, p. 232 and 187). Van Riper also discussed drill for carryover in a process he called *strengthening the new sound*: "A new sound must be strengthened before it can win the competition which the error provides" (Van Riper, 1954, p. 247).

A certain amount of drill seems necessary in almost every case, however drill has a dual nature. Drill can aid learning or detract from it depending upon how it is used. The old-timers said that we should not let it get boring: "One cannot overemphasize the fact that parrot-like drill is worse than useless" (Akin, 1958, p. 7). Van Riper said that drill should be varied, creative, and thoughtful to be beneficial to the carryover process. My experience agrees. Drill should be used to strengthen carryover, but it should not be overdone. Certainly drill should not be used as a sole method of treatment to promote carryover, but it has its place in the carryover process.

Drill, practice, and rehearsal can be accomplished in many ways depending upon the chronological age and cognitive level of the client. What makes this work interesting depends upon the client. It is left to the creative drive and natural teaching ability of each individual therapist to find ways that will encourage drill in their clients. For example:

- One client may drill like crazy to earn a few stickers to place on a worksheet.
- A second client may practice his speech for a solid thirty minutes if he can toss a ball into a hoop with every few trials.
- A third client may rehearse willingly if you play a game that involves throwing dice or spinning a wheel to determine the number of times he must practice.
- A fourth client may not drill unless you tell him NOT to say a particular sound or word—then he will keep saying it while you hold your ears and pretend that his production of the word is causing immense ear pain!

Perhaps the words practice and rehearsal soften the image that comes with the word drill. Obviously some clients need more practice to assure carryover, and others require less. It is the job of each speech-language pathologist to use direct clinical evidence to determine just how much rehearsal is necessary to assure carryover for each individual client. The amount of drill necessary cannot be prescribed. That depends upon the individual client's learning skills, his powers of habituation, and his motivation to change.

> *"The speech clinician, like the voice, golf, or basketball coach, must realize the fact that rehearsal can and must be viewed as an important and interesting*

component to improved performance. In so doing, we structure rehearsal to give it meaning, carefully evaluate its results, and enthusiastically reward its improvement" (Hoffman, Schuckers, and Daniloff, 1989, p. 248).

Positive and Negative Reinforcement

Anyone who has studied behavior modification understands that positive reinforcement tends to increase selected behaviors, negative reinforcement tends to decrease them, and intermittent variable ratio schedules are the best way to ensure that the subject will continue to be invested in the process. This means that we praise or reward our clients in response to the things they say correctly, we give clear feedback about utterances that are incorrect, and we sprinkle these comments throughout therapy in ways that are somewhat unpredictable to keep the client engaged.

Despite widespread knowledge of the positive effects of structured behavior management that arose in the 1960's, a change occurred in the 1970's. Teachers and therapists alike began to tell all children that they were doing well no matter what they did or how they performed. It was believed at the time that giving positive feedback all the time would encourage everyone equally. The student who made a brilliant painting of his house was told, "That's excellent!" and the child who put a few scratches on paper also was told the same thing. Sometimes the child with less skill needs this type of motivation. But my experience over three decades has been that this type of equalizing can cause problems. Kids who are doing poorly do not realize that they can and should try harder, and kids who are doing brilliantly do not get credit for the skill that they have. Clinicians who really want to move their clients toward carryover of speech skills must make sure that they are doling out both positive and negative reinforcement, and that they are giving these comments intermittently to keep the client invested in the process to the end.

Unfortunately, the everyone-is-a-winner philosophy still runs rampant in our culture. Some therapists today seem either to have forgotten, or were never exposed to, these most basic notions about behavior modification. Many therapists simply are giving out too much positive reinforcement. Some of these therapists even have abandoned the notion of correct/incorrect and shower clients with a neutral feedback statement such as, "That was a good try." A subject who receives neutral feedback like this does not know what to think about his performances. He is not being given any information about whether what he said was correct or incorrect. He comes to believe that everything he does is good, or he begins to think that he is making no progress whatsoever, or at the very least he gets confused. The self-evaluation a client must utilize during carryover stems from an ability to discriminate his own correct and incorrect performances, and that ability comes from clear boundaries set by the clinician through consistent positive and negative reinforcement. Inconsistent behavior management, too much positive reinforcement, and neutral statements drag out an articulation therapy program. One could almost guarantee that carryover with difficult clients will not be reached without the line between correct and incorrect productions firmly drawn.

Some young therapists today may not have experienced consistent positive and negative reinforcement themselves while they were in school, and they may view negative feedback as cruel. But it is not cruel to use negative feedback to help children learn. To understand this, take your mind into another area of endeavor. For example, consider what it would be like to take a cooking class. Would you like your instructor to give you specific information about what you were doing right and wrong, or would you just like the chef to tell you that you could do whatever you liked, and that each step you took was a good try? Common sense tells us that most of us like teachers to give clear signals of both a positive and negative nature so that we can learn quickly and efficiently. These things are absolutely critical for success in carryover.

Readers seeking more information on the effectiveness of positive and negative reinforcement are referred to almost any introductory psychology textbook. The reader also is referred to the discussion of behavior modification related directly to speech-language therapy in *Treatment Procedures in Communication Disorders* (Hegde, 1998).

Praise

Positive feedback usually involves some sort of praise. Garber, Garber, and Spizman gave specific advice about giving praise in their wonderful book for parents called *Good Behavior* (1990). Here are their five main suggestions with examples for articulation training:

- PRAISE BEHAVIOR AND NOT PERSONALITY: Don't say, "You are a good boy." Instead say, "You made a good L."
- USE SPECIFIC PRAISE: Don't say, "Good talking." Instead say, "You said *car* exactly right."
- PRAISE PROGRESS: Don't just say, "You did a good job today." Also say, "You are learning how to say Sh."
- PRAISE APPROPRIATELY: Don't say, "Okay… Yeah…" Instead say. "The second S you made was perfect. The first one wasn't that good."
- PRAISE IMMEDIATELY: Don't wait until the end of the session to tell the client he did well. Praise him after every few utterances.

75/25

My professors taught that 75% of each therapy session should contain work that is easy and familiar to the client, and only 25% should be new, unfamiliar, and challenging. My three decades of clinical experiences since then have affirmed this to be an excellent ratio.

Think about piano lessons in order to understand this ratio. A piano lesson rarely focuses entirely on things the student cannot do. Instead, most of the lesson is devoted to a rehearsal of those things the student already has been doing and can do fairly well. The teacher starts out the lesson with a statement like, "Show me what you have been working on this week." The teacher then tweaks the performance and adds a few new things to it. Over time the student gradually learns an increasingly larger repertoire of skills. Once in a while a lesson contains all new material to challenge the student and lift him to new heights. But the piano teacher knows that if every lesson is too hard, the student will get discouraged, may refuse to go to lessons, and may hate the piano for the rest of his life. The teacher wants to succeed with the student, and therefore provides an opportunity for him to feel successful by arranging the classes to contain more positive than negative experiences. We should do the same in articulation and phonological therapy. Such a ratio promotes carryover because each session reinforces skills already learned.

Therapists often ask what to do about a client who performs so poorly that he gets mostly negative feedback. When a client performs so poorly that the 75% correct performance level is not being reached, this simply means that the level of therapy is too high for him. In this case, we scale back and focus treatment on material that is easier for him. This is good for the client in several ways: It builds rapport, it helps the client feel excited about therapy, it builds his self-confidence, and it gives him courage to move forward.

Rewards

Rewards need to be given for progress in the carryover phase just like in all other phases of speech improvement. Small rewards should be given during the process, and the final reward needs to be significant since success in the carryover phase marks the end of the program. Small rewards include verbal praise, clapping, a hug, a big smile, a high-five, or a thumbs-up, and there are always the proverbial stars and stickers. A discussion of the therapist's pride in the child's accomplishments goes a long way as a short-term reward. The long-term reward has to be more meaningful because it is the reward for completing the program. The long-term reward might include a certificate of completion, a game, the honor of giving a graduation speech, a special birthday party, karate lessons, or a new bicycle. The client's personality should be taken into account when selecting the final reward for successful carryover, and don't forget to include the parents in this decision because they will be the ones paying for it. The fact that speech is finally over is enough of a reward for many kids.

Are Treasure Boxes Necessary?

Many therapists love to use a *Treasure Box* filled with little items that children can receive as a tangible reward for good work, and this certainly is a wonderful motivator for many children. But a treasure box is not required. Many therapists have no funds for such rewards, and some don't like to use them. I have never used a treasure box in more than thirty years of therapy, and perhaps this is because I am cheap. The truth is that I simply never got around to making one. I have always depended upon my ability to make clients feel proud about their progress as my primary means of reward at all levels of therapy, including the carryover phase. An open smile, a star drawn on the top of a paper, or a shout of "Perfect!" can do just as much or more than a little trinket that is broken or lost fifteen minutes after it is received. Tabor and Hambrecht (1997) felt that inexpensive rewards may not be that rewarding in the process of carryover. Engel et al (1966) said we should identify certain other adults that the client admires, and we should enlist their support as a giver of positive verbal rewards in the carryover phase: "One positive comment from the coach or clergyman may be worth many hours of the clinician's work and may provide reinforcement the clinician alone could never equal" (p. 231).

Plotting Progress

Old-time speech teachers emphasized that clients needed simple ways to understand their progress at all stages of therapy including the carryover phase: "Be sure he understands how far he has come and what his next task will be" (Powers, 1971, p. 899). Our predecessors often plotted a client's progress visually by using the image of a ladder, a stairway, or a thermometer. Graph paper also was used. For example, Van Riper and Irwin's *Voice and Articulation* (1958) contains a photograph of a boy standing next to a large speech thermometer drawn on a poster board labeled *Speech Meter* (p. 151). The thermometer is marked with lines, and each line tells of a stage of therapy from top to bottom as follows:

- I can make the correct sound all the time (top line of the thermometer)
- I can make the sound talking in the clinic
- I can make the sound reading
- I can make the sound at the end of words
- I can make the sound in the middle of words
- I can make the sound at the beginning of words
- I can make the sound with vowels
- I can make the sound by itself
- I know how to make the sound (bottom line of the thermometer)

The thermometer in this photograph is filled in all the way to the top, so I guess the boy has completed his program and has succeeded in the carryover phase. An old-fashioned idea like this seems corny today, yet we still work with children who can benefit from this type of concrete representation of their progress. Simple charts are used for adult projects even today, for example, I have seen thermometers used to mark progress for fundraising projects. A visual chart can be an essential part of a carryover program for some clients: "Any way of demonstrating, emphasizing, or illustrating improvement furthers [the] feeling of accomplishment" (Engel et al, 1966, p. 228).

SIMPLER CHARTING: A visual chart of progress can be made simpler for younger children. For example, have the client draw a happy face and a sad face. If he is working on L in the word *lady*, write "Wady" under the sad face, and write "Lady" under the happy face. Or use a picture of a puppy with the immature production, and use a picture of a mature dog with the correct production.

WORDS OF PROGRESS: Many therapists, including myself, make a big deal in therapy about what the clients "used to say" to help clients understand their own progress. For example: "You used to say, 'wabbit.' Now you say, 'rabbit.'" This is an excellent way to help children realize how far they have come. A video recording of the client before and after the change is an outstanding way to drive this idea home.

Punishment at Home

Parents need kind, safe, yet effective ways to punish their children for lack of attention to the process of carryover. Punishment is necessary during the very last stages of treatment when a client has complete control of his speech as long as he is thinking about it. Parents sometimes need a way to punish their child for not employing their new skill regularly. Faber and Mazlish (1980) is an excellent resource for parents in this regard. They discuss how to make effective punishment statements. Examples of ineffective statements re-written into effective ones are offered in Table 2. I have written the examples as they might be used with a 15-year-old who is working on R.

Baby-Sitting the Teen Client

Parents sometimes offer to baby-sit teens if they do not comply with rules, and this is a method we might adapt to carryover occasionally. For example, a mother reported that her teenage son developed a problem of tardiness to classes. One day the mother simply showed up at the high school and stood outside the class he was in. The son was shocked and embarrassed to see her

Table 2 – Ineffective vs. Effective Statements

Ineffective Statement	Alternative Effective Statement
CHASTISEMENT: "The dentist is going to think you are an idiot if you say R wrong during your visit."	POINT OUT A WAY TO BE HELPFUL: "It would help the dentist understand you if you say your R correctly while you are talking to him."
BELITTLING: "You are saying your R like a baby!"	EXPRESS STRONG DISAPPROVAL: "I don't like that old incorrect R. You can do better than that."
DEMAND: "Don't say R that way while grandma is here this afternoon!"	STATE YOUR EXPECTATIONS: "I expect you to say R correctly while grandma visits this afternoon."
THREAT: "If you say R wrong during dinner, I am going to take away your PlayStation!"	GIVE A CHOICE: "You can use the PlayStation after dinner if you use the sound correctly, but not if you don't. Your choice."
EMPTY THREAT: "I warned you! Every R sound was wrong during that ride. Now what am I supposed to do? Do I have to punish you?" [Followed by no punishment.]	TAKE ACTION AND ALLOW THE CHILD TO EXPERIENCE THE CONSEQUENCES OF HIS MISBEHAVIOR: "Ok. Every R sound was wrong during that ride. So I am putting away the PlayStation until tomorrow." [Followed by putting the item away.]

when he exited his class. When asked why she was there, she whispered to him that she wanted to make sure he got to his next class on time. She then walked him to his class. When they arrived at the door to the next class, she told him that she would be there every day to walk him from class to class if he needed any more help learning this important life skill. He got the message immediately and never was tardy again.

A simple offer to baby-sit like this might be sufficient to motivate an adolescent toward carryover. Speech-language pathologists can make such a suggestion in a non-threatening way by conveying the message that they are there to help the client in any way necessary, even by sitting with him during class or extracurricular activities. Of course the reason this method is designed specifically for teens is because younger children would love to have the SLP with them wherever they go. Typical adolescents will be much less open to the idea. A subtle suggestion that you are there to take care of his speech during other activities may be enough to jolt some of our most stubborn adolescents into paying attention to their own carryover needs.

Self-Imposed Punishment

Engel et al (1966) discussed the use of self-punishment in the carryover phase. The idea is for the client to make himself do something mildly unpleasant every time he catches himself making an error. For example, when he notices he has made an error, the client must untie and then re-tie his shoes, count to ten aloud, or snap his fingers 12 times. Determine a punishment that is age appropriate and gentle, but which grabs the child's attention and focuses it on his speech behavior. I have never used this idea myself because it never occurred to me, but it is an interesting idea that is worth trying with just the right client.

Goals for Carryover

Sheila Stull was kind enough to submit the following list of goals she uses during the carryover process. She has them organized into six levels:

1. Reading Aloud
    a. Reads aloud for 3 minutes with 90% accuracy.
    b. Reads aloud for 5 minutes with 90% accuracy.
    c. Reads aloud for 10 minutes with 90% accuracy.
2. Talking with the SLP
    a. Talks to SLP for 5 minutes using short answers with 90% accuracy.
    b. Talks to SLP for 10 minutes using short answers with 90% accuracy.
    c. Talks to SLP for 15 minutes using short answers with 90% accuracy.
3. Conversation with SLP
    a. Has a 5-minute conversation with SLP with 90% accuracy.
    b. Has a 10-minute conversation with SLP with 90% accuracy.
    c. Has a 15-minute conversation with SLP with 90% accuracy.
4. Conversation with a peer
    a. Has a 10-minute conversation with a friend in speech room with 90% accuracy.
    b. Has a 15-minute conversation with a friend in speech room with 90% accuracy.
5. Good articulation with teacher
    a. Uses good articulation (teacher checks ALL or MOST OF THE TIME on a score sheet) for 4/5 days in 1 class for 1 week.
    b. Uses good articulation (teacher checks ALL or MOST OF THE TIME on a score sheet) for 4/5 days in 2 classes for 1 week.
    c. Uses good articulation (3 checks ALL or MOST OF THE TIME on a score sheet) for 4/5 days in three classes for 1 week.
    d. Uses good articulation (teacher checks ALL or MOST OF THE TIME on a score sheet) for 4/5 days in 4 classes for 1 week.
    e. Uses good articulation (teacher checks ALL or MOST OF THE TIME on a score sheet) for 4/5 days in all classes for 1 week.
6. Good articulation with parents
    a. Uses good articulation (parent checks ALL or MOST OF THE TIME on a score sheet)

for 10 minutes with parents for 1 week.

b. Uses good articulation (parent checks ALL or MOST OF THE TIME on a score sheet) for 20 minutes with parents for 1 week.

c. Uses good articulation (parent checks ALL or MOST OF THE TIME on a score sheet) for 30 minutes with parents for 1 week.

d. Uses good articulation (parent checks ALL or MOST OF THE TIME on a score sheet) for 60 minutes with parents for 1 week.

e. Uses good articulation (parent checks ALL or MOST OF THE TIME on a score sheet) from 7 to 9 p.m. for 1 week.

f. Uses good articulation (parent checks ALL or MOST OF THE TIME on a score sheet) all the time with parents for 2 weeks.

Behavior Modification Program for Cognitive Deficit

McLean (1970) proposed a *stimulus shift program* for carryover based on behavior modification designed for children with cognitive deficit. They utilized a stimulus-response-reinforcement paradigm and organized the program into four stimulus conditions that they found helpful for stimulating carryover:

1. ECHOIC STIMULUS CONDITION: The client imitates the therapist's model of the target word.
2. TEXTUAL/PICTURE STIMULUS CONDITION: The child responds to a presentation of a picture of the word.
3. TEXTUAL/PRINTED WORD STIMULUS CONDITION: The client responds to the presentation of the printed word. This stage is omitted if the child cannot read.
4. INTRAVERBAL STIMULUS CONDITION: The child responds by completing a sentence using one of his training words.

*

Chapter 6 Summary

The Role of Behavior Modification in Carryover

- Carryover is possible when clients are engaged in a consistent behavior modification program.
- Speech-language pathologists must have a clear goal in mind, and this idea must be transmitted to the client.
- Most therapists view practice, drill, and rehearsal as important methods of speech habituation.
- Clients should receive positive reinforcement in response to the things they say correctly, and they should be given clear feedback about utterances that are incorrect.
- Rewards and punishments are sprinkled throughout therapy in ways that are somewhat unpredictable. This keeps clients engaged.
- A client who gets too much positive reinforcement, or who hears too many neutral phrases about his performances may get confused. This interferes with the long-term carryover goal.
- Positive feedback usually involves some sort of praise.
- Articulation therapy can be equated to weekly piano lessons. Most lessons are devoted in large measure to performance of skills the student can do fairly well.
- Rewards need to be given for progress in the carryover phase just like in all other phases of speech improvement.
- A treasure box is a fun addition but not a requirement of an effective behavior management program. An open smile or a word of praise from a favored adult can do just as much or more than a tangible reward.
- Simple charts are used to help clients monitor their own progress.
- Parents need safe yet effective ways to punish their children for lack of attention to the process of carryover at home.
- Clients can administer their own negative reinforcement outside of treatment for carryover.

Chapter 7

Conversational Speech in the Carryover Process

"So easily does the careless speaker fall from grace after all his errors have been nicely corrected."

– Richard Borden and Alvin Busse, 1925

When I was a young therapist, I used to think that conversation was something one stuck onto the end of a good articulation program. I thought of conversation as an afterthought, something insignificant and bothersome, and something we had to force ourselves to do in order to finish up a program. I was wrong. Three decades of working directly with children has taught me that conversational work is something that should be integrated into therapy from the first day. A lack of change in articulatory performance during the demands of conversational speech may signal that therapy is not directed toward conversational speech. Elbert et al (1991) demonstrated that many children do carryover speech skills without working directly on conversation, but not all of them did. Some clients need to work directly on conversation —

> *"It is not unusual for parents or teachers to report little change in articulation patterns at school or home, while the speech-language pathologist is aware of adequate progress in speech sessions. Frequently this is based on the fact that modification of errors has not occurred in conversational speech"* (Bosley, 1981, p. 20).

Once I began to pull all my skills together and work at a conversational level right from the start of therapy, my clients began to progress much more quickly. Working at the conversational level is a process of putting every type of facilitation technique together into one package.

Traditional Ideas About Conversation

There is a widespread misconception today that our predecessors worked only on non-functional drill of phonemes, syllables, and words, and that they did not work on functional communication and conversational skills. For example, in an article about practice versus functional communication, one modern author called prior decades "the days when speech-language therapy was routinely conducted in sterile, non-communicative contexts" (Kamhi, 2000, p. 185). This is an erroneous belief that has been espoused time and again. It simply is not true. Admonitions to work on functional communication and conversational speech are found all throughout historic books on articulation therapy, even in some of our earliest texts. Working directly on conversation is a procedure that has been part of articulation therapy since the beginning. Here are a few examples that span the decades:

- *1912*: "In a group of two people, talk on assigned topics of conversation, with material prepared beforehand. Then with three people, and so on, gradually increasing the number in the group. Gradually bring in strangers" (Scripture, 1912, p. 222).
- *1937*: "The drills are presented without exception in the form of motivated games and devices [activities]. The game and [activity] approach not only stimulates interest but also provides a more nearly normal speech situation ...[These games and activities] assist in bridging the gap between formal repetition of speech exercises and the carryover into spontaneous speaking" (Nemoy and Davis, 1937, p. xi).
- *1939*: "One of the most important steps in the treatment of both articulatory and voice disorders is getting the child to use the new sound consistently in his daily conversations. It is not enough merely to teach the child how to make the correct sound; he must follow a systematic program of effecting the transition into casual speech" (Van Riper, 1939, p. 257).
- *1965*: "When the child incorporates his sound into words easily, he is ready to begin the transfer to his everyday speech. His teacher, correctionist, and parents need to provide as many speaking situations as possible. At this stage the teacher is as important as the correctionist, for she can set up situations wherein the child has many speaking and reading opportunities to incorporate his newly acquired sounds ... Creative activities, including both puppetry and creative drama, encourage children to talk ... Other situations for just plain talk arise spontaneously" (Eisenson and Ogilvie, 1965, p. 247-248).
- *1981*: "Carryover will proceed from limited, highly structured speaking situations ... It will then build gradually to less limited and less highly structured situations in the training room and in the home until at last it is achieved for spontaneous speech" (Bosley, 1981, p. 109).

Van Riper

Most modern articulation and phonological textbooks today support Van Riper's advice about working on conversation. He suggested that conversational speech should start with definite periods at school and at home during which the client will be corrected on each misarticulated word. He said that these times should be very short at first, and length should increase over time. Following Van Riper, Bosley (1981) suggested that the level of difficulty of individual conversations should be viewed in light of the child's age, temperament, and interests. She also said that conversations should develop from least to most interesting to the child. Bosley arranged a hierarchy of conversation from least interesting to most interesting along these lines:

1. Speak to one person only, probably the mother.
2. Speak on subjects void of great interest: the weather, what clothes the child will wear tomorrow, what he might like for breakfast, and so forth.
3. Speak with the mother and one other person, probably the father, on similar topics.
4. Look at books and talk about the pictures.
5. Play games where comments are fairly routine, for example, "Your turn," "You can't move there," "I'm ahead of you," and so forth.
6. Retell a story.
7. Talk about a day at school if it has been routine.
8. Review an incident from the day before that was interesting.
9. Ask questions of the mother or another family member.
10. Talk about an especially interesting television program or movie.
11. Plan an exciting weekend.
12. Try to convince a parent that permission should be given for something special.
13. Argue with adults.
14. Argue with peers.

Dos and Don'ts of Conversation

The traditional view is that conversation follows work on words, phrases, sentences, paragraphs, and other reading material. I use this method, of course, but I have developed what I believe to be a better approach to conversation. It is a way that conversational work can be integrated into therapy right from the first day of treatment. The rest of this chapter will be devoted to my process of using conversational speech to promote carryover. Just like Van Riper, this information comes from many years of clinical experimentation with a wide variety of clients. The following are lessons my professors, my clients, and my observations of the human experience, have taught me about how to work conversation into treatment. These are the *Dos and Don'ts* of conversational work:

1. Don't hog the conversation. Conversation is a two-way process. Let the child talk.
2. Don't ask too many questions. This encourages kids to make single-word responses.
3. Make statements for your turn. This encourages the client to make his own original statements.
4. Make short remarks for your turn. Pontificating adults bore kids.
5. Pause after your remark. This bounces the conversational ball back to the client.
6. Imitate the child's comment back to him for your turn periodically. This lets him know that you are listening to his every word. It encourages him to keep talking. Don't do this too much, and don't do it if it bothers the client.
7. Don't assume that the child can abstract the idea of speaking correctly just because you are doing so. He needs to know exactly what is going on. Tell him. Don't assume he will understand that this is what he is supposed to do without direct instruction.
8. Start by talking about the target phoneme itself. Make the target phoneme the subject of the conversation. Get this started by asking, "Why did you come here?"

9. Stay on topic, but be sensitive to the child's topic leads.
10. Have two topics running simultaneously. Let the first be the target phoneme and the second be of the client's interest. For example, talk about the S sounds in dinosaur names.
11. Place less emphasis on the phoneme topic and more emphasis on the child's topic over time.
12. Ellocute. Show your client how to speak with clarity and distinction.
13. Speak at a child's rate. Speak in the same number of words per minute as the client. Adjust rate a little faster or slower to see which way facilitates more client output during conversations.
14. Don't make your speech sugarcoated and fake. Find your adult voice and use it. Older children usually dismiss the advice of adults who speak to them in a cute voice. They say, "She treats me like a baby."
15. Sprinkle age-appropriate slang into the dialogue, but don't use too much because the kids will think you are weird and trying too hard. Ask the client what certain slang words and phrases mean. This allows them to see that you are interested in them and their generation.
16. Don't use curse words even if they are a part of the popular culture. Set a higher professional standard. Children respect this deep down inside.
17. Allow time periodically for the child to ramble on about his favorite topic without correction. This allows him to speak freely to you. It will assure him that he can talk about whatever he wants with you. This has a tremendous psychological impact on him. He will begin to speak to you freely, and you may even become his favorite conversational partner. This will give you ample opportunity to work on conversational skills all the time. The impact on conversation outside of the therapy room will be tremendous.
18. Use conversation time to monitor carryover and to discover the client's favorite topics.

Sample Dialogues

The best way to understand conversational work is to watch and listen to dialogues. The next best thing to watching and listening to dialogues is to read them. The three conversations that comprise the rest of this chapter take place during therapy. The dialogues are between a speech-language pathologist and an adolescent boy with a simple frontal lisp. The dialogues demonstrate how carryover can be promoted at all levels of treatment. The samples represent three basic levels of therapy:

1. DIALOGUE A: The first dialogue represents early therapy in which the client is just performing isolated phonemes consistently. The therapist is embedding isolated sound productions into a dialogue, and she is pushing him on to a few word productions.
2. DIALOGUE B: The second dialogue represents therapy a little while later, when the client is at the word level. Now the therapist picks out a key word, and she structures the dialogue around it. The therapist tries to get the client to say the key word as many times as possible within the dialogue. She ignores all other words that contain the target.
3. DIALOGUE C: The third dialogue takes place much later, when the client now should be taking full control of his correct phoneme. The therapist is prodding him to say it

correctly throughout the entire dialogue by blocking his messages if he says the sound wrong.

Key to The Dialogues

- The symbol "sss" represents the phoneme spoken in isolation.
- The symbol "ssssssssss" represents a long prolongation of the phoneme.
- The symbol "Ess" represents the naming of the alphabet letter.
- A dash (—) indicates a pause.
- Actions are noted in brackets. For example, [Smiles.]
- The right-hand column gives a brief analysis of the techniques being employed by the therapist.

Dialogue A: Phoneme as Subject

The earliest dialogues in the unfolding sequence of articulation therapy should be about the target phoneme itself. Treat the target phoneme as the subject of the conversation. Talk about

Dialogue A – Phoneme as Subject

Speaker	Spoken Utterance	Techniques Employed
THERAPIST	That Ess was perfect.	Giving positive reinforcement
CLIENT	[Smiles.]	
THERAPIST	I did not know you could say it so well.	Creating a positive atmosphere
CLIENT	[Silence.]	
THERAPIST	Now… why are you coming here?	Getting client focused on purpose of therapy
CLIENT	To learn my Ess? [Spoken incorrectly.]	
THERAPIST	Oh, yea. To learn your Ess. Do you think you could say it five times in a row?	Ignoring the client's error on S because it was embedded in a sentence. Encouraging drill
CLIENT	Maybe.	
THERAPIST	Let's try. Listen to mine — Sss-sss-sss-sss-sss. Now you do it.	Modeling the isolated phoneme

continued on page 78

Speaker	Spoken Utterance	Techniques Employed
CLIENT	Sss-sss-sss-sss-sss. [Spoken correctly.]	
THERAPIST	Very nice. Do you think they were correct?	Giving positive reinforcement Requesting auditory self-discrimination
CLIENT	I think so.	
THERAPIST	Yes. They were perfect. Very nice… Ess is a weird letter. It's all curvy. Let me show you how I like to write mine. [Writes a fancy letter S.]	Giving positive reinforcement Leading into a break from production Leading into a spelling task
CLIENT	Cool.	
THERAPIST	That's a curly sssssssss.	Modeling phoneme at end of a phrase with prolongation
CLIENT	I like it.	
THERAPIST	Say, A curly sssssssss.	Modeling phoneme at end of a phrase with prolongation
CLIENT	A curly sssssssss.	
THERAPIST	Excellent. I like to make my letter all fancy and curly. Do you want to try it? Here… [Hands client a red marker.] Make it in red.	Giving positive reinforcement Leading into spelling
CLIENT	[Writes several curly letters, each one getting curlier.]	
THERAPIST	Wow. Those are very curly. Do you know any words that start with the sound sssssssss?	Giving positive reinforcement Stimulating cognition Modeling target phoneme with emphasis Pushing on to next level of performance — words with initial S

continued on page 79

Speaker	Spoken Utterance	Techniques Employed
CLIENT	Yea, like, snow. [Sound spoken incorrectly.]	
THERAPIST	Say, Ssssssssssnow. And keep your tongue in the right place.	Modeling with emphasis Reiterating instructions
CLIENT	Ssssssssssnow. [Correct production.]	
THERAPIST	I think that was right. Check in the mirror. Say, Ssssssssssnow.	Eliciting the client's visual discrimination Modeling with emphasis again
CLIENT	[Looks in mirror.] Ssssssssssnow.	
THERAPIST	Was it correct?	Asking for client's discrimination
CLIENT	Yea. I think so.	
THERAPIST	Why was it correct?	Stimulating cognition
CLIENT	Because I kept my tongue in and the sound came out the middle? [This is repetition of the instructions that have been drilled into his head for the past two weeks.]	
THERAPIST	Yes. Because you kept your tongue in and the sound came out the middle.	Giving positive reinforcement Reiterating the instructions
CLIENT	[Silence.]	
THERAPIST	Perfect. You know, Ess is very hard to say for some kids.	Giving positive reinforcement Giving empathy
CLIENT	Really?	
THERAPIST	Yep. It's one of the hardest sounds in the world.	Giving empathy Providing information
CLIENT	I think it's easy. [Target phoneme spoken incorrectly.]	

continued on page 80

Speaker	Spoken Utterance	Techniques Employed
THERAPIST	Really? Let me hear you say it again…	Ignoring incorrect utterance beyond current level of therapy Cueing for another production at his level of production
CLIENT	Sssssssss. [Spoken correctly.]	
THERAPIST	Yep. That's exactly right. You kept your tongue inside. Now, let's think. What other words have Sssssssss? … Do you know any words that have Ess at the end?	Giving positive reinforcement Reiterating instructions Modeling phoneme Stimulating cognition Pushing on to next level of performance — words with final /s/
CLIENT	Ummm… yea, ummm… mouse. [Spoken correctly.]	
THERAPIST	Mouse! Very nice. You thought about it, and you came up with one. And do you know what?	Giving positive reinforcement Piquing the client's curiosity
CLIENT	What?	
THERAPIST	You said it perfectly.	Giving delayed positive reinforcement
CLIENT	[Smiles.]	
THERAPIST	Say, mousssssssssse, mousssssssssse, mousssssssssse. Three times.	Modeling target word multiple times Emphasizing target phoneme with prolongation
CLIENT	Mousssssssssse, mousssssssssse, mousssssssssse. [Said correctly.]	
THERAPIST	Perfect again!	Giving positive reinforcement
CLIENT	[Smiles.]	

continued on page 81

Speaker	Spoken Utterance	Techniques Employed
THERAPIST	I didn't realize how smart you are!	Ego-building
CLIENT	I think I am kind of smart. Not too smart, though. [Spoken incorrectly.]	
THERAPIST	Well, smart enough to figure out Ess. Now what should we do? Oh — How about another word that ends in Ess. What about Bus? Does that end in Ess?	Ignoring incorrect sounds beyond current level Stimulating cognition Stimulating auditory discrimination

this phoneme, the way it sounds, the way it's made, and its corresponding orthographic symbol or symbols. Integrate simple syllable and word productions into the dialogue to carry the work from the isolated phoneme to the next steps of therapy.

Dialogue B: Key Word as Subject

We can move the dialogue ahead by focusing on single words. Most clients have trouble incorporating their new skill into everyday conversation because that requires the client to do two things at once: He must talk freely and monitor himself at the same time. This can be difficult. At first the mind has to switch back-and-forth between these two skills. I have found that the best way to do this is to structure the dialogue around one key word. That way, the conversation can get very complex, but the production the child is keeping track of within the conversation is very simple.

Dialogue B – Key Word as Subject

Speaker	Spoken Utterance	Techniques Employed
THERAPIST	The word soup is interesting to me. I like — soup.	Selecting a key word Modeling the key word Pausing before the key word to emphasize the target phoneme
CLIENT	Yea, me too.	

continued on page 82

Speaker	Spoken Utterance	Techniques Employed
THERAPIST	I think my favorite is split pea — soup.	Modeling the key word Pausing before the key word to emphasize the target phoneme Urging participation by picking an example the client probably will not like
CLIENT	Blaaaaaa. I like my grandma's. [Phoneme S spoken incorrectly.]	
THERAPIST	Your grandma's what?	Ignoring error on word beyond the topic and the child's current production capability Prodding client to use key word spontaneously
CLIENT	My grandma's soup. [Spoken incorrectly.]	
THERAPIST	Did you say it correctly?	Prodding client's own discrimination
CLIENT	Huh?	
THERAPIST	Soup. When you said, "My grandma's ssssssssssoup." Did you say soup the way we have been practicing?	Modeling key word Prolonging target phoneme in key word Prodding client's own discrimination
CLIENT	I don't know. [Shrugs.]	
THERAPIST	Oh. Well, say it again. And think about it.	Accepting the inevitable Prodding discrimination again
CLIENT	Say what?	
THERAPIST	Say, "My grandma's — soup."	Giving a direct instruction Modeling target word Pausing before target
CLIENT	My grandma's soup.	

continued on page 83

Speaker	Spoken Utterance	Techniques Employed
THERAPIST	How was that one? Did you say — sssssssssssoup — correctly?	Prodding discrimination again Modeling target word Prolonging target Pausing before and after target
CLIENT	Yes?	
THERAPIST	Yes! You said it perfectly.	Giving positive reinforcement
CLIENT	[Smiles.]	
THERAPIST	Okay. Now what were you saying about your grandma's — sssssssssssoup?	Continuing the dialogue Pausing before target Prolonging target
CLIENT	I like it.	
THERAPIST	Say, "I like my grandma's — sssssssssssoup."	Modeling target word in sentence Pausing before target Prolonging target
CLIENT	I like my grandma's sssssssss-soup.	
THERAPIST	Very nice. Now, why? Why do you like it?	Giving positive reinforcement Continuing the dialogue
CLIENT	Oh man, it's the best. [S spoken incorrectly.]	
THERAPIST	What kind is it?	Ignoring error Continuing the dialogue
CLIENT	Chicken noodle.	
THERAPIST	Say, chicken noodle — sssssssssssoup.	Modeling word in phrase Emphasizing the key word Pausing before target Prolonging target
CLIENT	Chicken noodle sssssssssssoup.	

continued on page 84

Speaker	Spoken Utterance	Techniques Employed
THERAPIST	Very nice. I think you said—sssssssssssoup—correctly that time. Did you?	Giving positive reinforcement Modeling target word Pausing before target Prolonging target Requesting discrimination
CLIENT	Ummmmm…	
THERAPIST	Oh no! You forgot to listen to yourself again. [Laughs.]	Teasing to build rapport Reminding of instruction Encouraging self-monitoring
CLIENT	Oh, yea. [Laughs.]	
THERAPIST	Now, here's the thing. You will only fix your Ess if you listen. How can you remember to listen to yourself when you say soup?	Giving instruction Reminding about self-monitor-ing Eliciting the client's own ideas about carryover
CLIENT	I need a note.	
THERAPIST	A note?	Following client lead
CLIENT	Yea. When my mom wants to remember something she puts a note on the refrigerator. [All target sounds spoken incor-rectly.]	
THERAPIST	You know what? I do that too. When I have to remember sssssssssssomething, I write myssssssssssself a note. Sssssssssso, should we write a note?	Ignoring errors Accepting client's idea Modeling words Prolonging targets
CLIENT	Yea.	
THERAPIST	What should it sssssssssssay?	Eliciting more contributions from client Modeling word Prolonging target

continued on page 85

Speaker	Spoken Utterance	Techniques Employed
CLIENT	Soup. [Spoken incorrectly.]	
THERAPIST	Just sssssssssoup?	Ignoring error Modeling target word Prolonging targets
CLIENT	Yea, cause if it says soup I will remember the right way. [Spoken incorrectly.]	
THERAPIST	Okay. Here's a post-it.	Ignoring error Encouraging spelling
CLIENT	[Writes *S-O-U-P*.]	
THERAPIST	What did you write on it?	Cueing target word
CLIENT	Sssssssssoup!	
THERAPIST	Wow! How well did you say that one?	Giving positive reinforcement Prodding auditory discrimination Drawing attention to correct production
CLIENT	I think that one was good.	
THERAPIST	Yes! That one was perfect. What else do you do at your grandma's?	Giving positive reinforcement Continuing the dialogue

Dialogue C: Blocking the Message

A new strategy begins later in therapy in order to push the client into dialogues that require more effort and control on his part. Up until now, the therapist has guided the client carefully by using a wide variety of facilitation techniques within the dialogue. The therapist has modeled, emphasized, instructed, and so forth. To move the client ahead into the final stages of dialogue means to remove most of this help. It means forcing the client to use his skills spontaneously by blocking his ability to get his message across. It also means speaking directly about the process of self-repair, comparing and contrasting words, trying to see if he can catch you speaking incorrectly yourself, and getting him to repair your errors.

The idea is that the ultimate reason for a client to change is so he can get his message across. If the message gets across, there is no reason to change. So the therapist has to block the message. If the message does not get across, then the client has to think about what he can do to get it across. The client has learned most of the tools he needs to do this in therapy already. Now he is going to be expected to use them. This next conversation takes us to this level. Notice that the SLP makes the client work hard to get his message across, and then she begins a discussion of reminders that may help him.

It is important to note that blocking messages would be a very cruel way to work if the client did not have advanced control over his correct production and his error. When the client is ready, however, teachers, parents, and other adults can be taught to block messages by acting confused when the client mispronounces. Contributor Margaret Combs teaches adults that when they hear the client produce a sound incorrectly in spontaneous speech, they are to gently and politely block clients' messages by saying, "Excuse me?" Margaret teaches her students that "Excuse me" actually means, "Oops, you made a speech sound error. Fix it please." After the client repairs his error in the conversation, she has the adult say, "Thank you." This signals that the client repaired correctly. Margaret obtains her client's permission before she initiates this procedure with other adults.

Dialogue C – Blocking the Message

Speaker	Spoken Utterance	Techniques Employed
THERAPIST	That sounds like a good idea.	Continuing the dialogue
CLIENT	Yea, my dad said we could do it next thummer. (He means, *summer*.)	
THERAPIST	Next thummer? What's a thummer?	Blocking transmission of the message Imitating the client's error back to him to jar his awareness
CLIENT	No, not thummer. Thummer.	
THERAPIST	Thummer?	Blocking transmission of the message Imitating the client's error back to him to jar his awareness Forcing the client to come up with a solution
CLIENT	Sssssssssummer!	

continued on page 87

Speaker	Spoken Utterance	Techniques Employed
THERAPIST	Oh! Sssssssssummer! I didn't know WHAT you were talking about. I was trying to figure out what a "thummer" was. I thought it was something you did with your thumbs. [Smiles.]	Letting the message get through Reinforcing correct sound in target word Modeling both the correct and incorrect productions Prolonging the target Enlisting minimal pair comparisons
CLIENT	[Laughs.] No… Sssssssssummer.	
THERAPIST	Oh, so your dad said you could go there next sssssssssummer.	Continuing the dialogue Modeling correct phoneme in target word Prolonging target
CLIENT	Yea.	
THERAPIST	But why not now? Can't you go right now?	Continuing the dialogue
CLIENT	No. I don't think tho. I gueth they're not open.	
THERAPIST	I couldn't understand you.	Blocking the message because of the errors
CLIENT	I ssssssssssaid, "I guesssssssss they're not open."	
THERAPIST	Oh. They're not open in the winter?	Letting the message get through because he repaired his error Continuing the dialogue
CLIENT	No, only in thummer.	
THERAPIST	Huh?	Blocking transmission of the message
CLIENT	I mean, summer! Man! I keep forgetting!	

continued on page 88

Speaker	Spoken Utterance	Techniques Employed
THERAPIST	Oh, yea. Sssssssssummer. Sssssssssometimes that's a hard one to remember. Does your whole family go?	Allowing transmission Expressing empathy Continuing the dialogue
CLIENT	Yea.	
THERAPIST	Now, let's see if I can remember your brothers' names… There's Jathon… [She means Jason.]	Adding more target words to the conversation Challenging client's auditory attention and discrimination
CLIENT	Jasssssssssson.	
THERAPIST	Oh, yea. It has an Ess… Jasssssssssson. I was thinking that it was spelled J-A-T-H-O-N.	Comparing correct and error productions Prolonging the model Bringing in the spelling cues
CLIENT	No. An Ess.	
THERAPIST	Okay. J-A-S-O-N. Jason. [Spelling.] And, let's see… Mark?	Continuing the dialogue
CLIENT	Yea.	
THERAPIST	And, um who else?	Encouraging client participation in dialogue
CLIENT	Sam.	
THERAPIST	Sam?	Questioning his production
CLIENT	Yea, Sam.	
THERAPIST	I thought his name was Tham.	Comparing old and new productions
CLIENT	No. That's the way I used to say it.	
THERAPIST	How?	Forcing the client to produce the old error
CLIENT	Tham.	

continued on page 89

Speaker	Spoken Utterance	Techniques Employed
THERAPIST	Tham?	Modeling the old error
CLIENT	Yea.	
THERAPIST	How do you say it now?	Honoring client's new skill Letting him take the lead in using the new skill
CLIENT	Sssssssssam.	
THERAPIST	Oh yea, Sssssssssam. That is a lot better.	Allowing the client to become teacher
CLIENT	[Silent.]	
THERAPIST	I just realized something… They don't sound the same at all. Tham… Sam… Tham… Sam…	Putting descriptive words to the comparison Modeling the differences Using minimal pairs to highlight the differences
CLIENT	I know.	
THERAPIST	I can't believe you used to say it that way.	Praising his new ability
CLIENT	I know.	
THERAPIST	You are getting so good at this.	Ego-building
CLIENT	Thankth.	
THERAPIST	Thankth? [Looking surprised.]	Imitating the client's error
CLIENT	Man!	
THERAPIST	We need a way to help you remember this…	Enlisting client input for carry-over ideas
CLIENT	Yea…	
THERAPIST	What do you think?	Enlisting client input for carry-over ideas
CLIENT	Huh?	

continued on page 90

Speaker	Spoken Utterance	Techniques Employed
THERAPIST	What will you need to remember this every time?	Enlisting client input for carryover ideas
CLIENT	I don't know... Maybe I could just remember.	
THERAPIST	I don't know... That doesn't seem to be working all the time. You need a reminder.	Encouraging client to think through the problem
CLIENT	Like what?	
THERAPIST	Some kids use a dot.	Suggestion of a carryover reminder
CLIENT	A dot?	
THERAPIST	Yea. Some kids put a dot on their finger. A tiny dot. Like this. [Puts a dot on her own finger.]	Explanation of method Demonstration
CLIENT	[Watches. Puts a dot on his own finger.]	
THERAPIST	There. Now every time you see the dot you will be reminded to say your sound correctly.	
CLIENT	Cool.	

*

Chapter 7 Summary

Conversational Speech in the Carryover Process

- Conversational work can be integrated into therapy from the first day.
- Conversation is not an afterthought. It is an integral part of therapy.
- Conversation has been recommended as a part of articulation therapy since the inception of the profession.
- Van Riper recommends that conversational speech should start with definite periords during which the client should be corrected on each misarticulated word.
- Marshalla has proposed a different way to work on conversation in this chapter.
- Early conversations embed isolated sound productions and push the client on to a few word productions.
- Key words are used in conversations when a client is at the word level.
- At the word level, the therapist tries to get the client to say the target word as many times as possible within the dialogue. All other words that contain the target phoneme are ignored.
- A client should take full control of his correct phoneme in later dialogues. The therapist prods correct words all throughout the dialogue.
- Blocking messages is used to force change in mature dialogues.
- Later dialogues contain instruction about reminders.

Chapter 8

Personality, Emotion, and Attitude in Carryover

> *"At all stages, articulation therapy must be oriented psychotherapeutically. Attention must be given, not only to the development of accurate articulation but also to the individual's security and pleasure in speaking, to improvement of his communicative attitudes and habits, and to his motivation for personal speech improvement."*
>
> – Margaret Hall Powers, 1971

This chapter presents a discussion of the roles of personality, emotion, and attitude in the carryover process. A variety of subjects will be explored including personality domains, fluctuating emotions, building rapport, giving encouragement, developing client willingness or determination to change, dealing with client fear of change, handling client embarrassment, and other topics relevant to the carryover process. Virtually none of these ideas have been tested in terms of their effectiveness in articulation therapy. These are methods adapted to speech therapy from other areas of therapeutic intervention.

Attitude Adjustment

A client's *attitude* about therapy is his outlook, stance, position, mind-set, or opinion about therapy. Some clients enter therapy with a positive attitude, of course, and this contributes right away to a positive environment for carryover. Traditional therapists often wrote about the role that a positive attitude plays in carryover: "The client's desire to improve his speech is a powerful force in obtaining carryover" (Engel et al, 1966, p. 228). I am reminded here of a five-year-old girl with a distorted R. When asked why she came to my room that very first day, she sat up very straight and declared, "I can't say my R! I need to learn to say my R!" Now there's a girl who has a great attitude and will carry herself through the entire program with very little additional encouragement from the SLP.

Unfortunately not all clients are as motivated as that little girl. Some of our clients have a very poor attitude about speech correction due to feelings of hopelessness, unconcern, or distrust. Van Riper advised us to be concerned about psychological factors in all our clients: "A certain amount of psychotherapy is employed by every speech correctionist with every case"

(Van Riper, 1947, p. 52). He said that the methods of psychotherapy we use to help adjust client attitude range from simple suggestions to profound psychoanalysis. Van Riper had a problem of fluency, and I am sure he thought about this aspect of speech remediation very carefully. He suggested that whether the psychological aspect of treatment is light or plentiful, the plan should include at least the following:

1. Help the client understand his problem. Convince him he has a problem if necessary.
2. Let the client express his repressed feelings.
3. Help the client organize and carry out a campaign to increase his social assets and eliminate his social shortcomings.
4. Help the client eliminate or minimize the penalties he imposes upon himself because of his speech defect.
5. Help the client develop attitudes about his speech that will free him. Help him develop a reason to change.

Rapport

The writers of traditional articulation therapy always insisted that establishing rapport was the first critical step in the speech remediation process, and from this we can assume that rapport also is necessary to build carryover skill. *Rapport* is a trusting bond or a psychological connection between people. In our case, rapport is a trusting bond between the client and the therapist. The more connected the client feels with his speech-language pathologist, the more the clinician's ideas about carryover become central to the client's very existence. Difficulty in the carryover process can be due to a breakdown in rapport. It is the work of the treating speech-language pathologist to discover how to establish rapport with each and every client so that articulation therapy can succeed through to the stage of carryover. To have rapport with a client does not mean that the SLP and client become best friends. It means that the two have a close and harmonious working relationship in which they communicate well and understand each other's feelings or ideas. A therapist's personality and natural teaching ability plays a huge role in building rapport. Therapists use humor, a caring attitude, positive reinforcement, a genuine interest in the client, and many other factors to build rapport.

Encouragement

It has been said that correction does much, but that encouragement does more. Encouragement is emotional backup. It means to give a person support, confidence, or hope. Most clients need some level of encouragement to move into and through the carryover process. We encourage our clients in order to inspire them in a forward direction. Speech-language pathologists can encourage clients to use new speech skills outside the speech room just as a coach might encourage a team to play well in the next game. Simple messages of support made by someone who cares can contribute much to a client's carryover process: "You can do it! I know you can. I can't wait to hear how you do on your next speech assignment." Enlist others in this process, too. Use any adult the child admires, for example, a coach, teacher, parent, custodian, scout leader, clergy, neighbor, doctor, or dentist. Also use supportive and enthusiastic older children who have achieved success in their own process of speech remediation.

Pressure

Sometimes the best thing we can do for carryover is to take the pressure off. Pressure to perform perfectly may be the very cause of failed carryover. Some of these kids are crumbling under excessive pressure. I have seen many children cry in therapy because a parent is telling them to "Get this over with!" or "Do it!" Clients who come to therapy under a great deal of pressure may need to realize that learning a new speech sound is no big deal. Tell the client that he will figure it out eventually. Tell him that he may be ready for this work now, or next month, or next year, and that it doesn't matter either way. Express calm patience, and give parents gentle but firm advice to back off. Help these parents see that their pressure is not serving the child well. I usually say, "I am hoping we can lighten things up a little so he doesn't feel so much pressure about this. He is trying really hard, and if we back up a little I think he will have more success." On occasion I have acknowledged to the client privately that his parents are overly worried. I say, "Don't worry. Everything is okay. You will be able to do this just fine. You just need a little help. This is no big deal. I'm going to talk to your parents about this."

Emotional Noise

A client's emotional state can be an important part of the carryover process. *Emotion* is "a natural instinctive state of mind derived from one's circumstances, mood, or relationships with others" (Jewell and Abate, 2001, p. 557). The term *feeling* is commonly used for emotion. The problem with emotions or feelings is that they vary from moment to moment. Emotions sway depending upon the situation and a person's reaction to it. Emotions change with conditions, atmosphere, humor, temper, status, position, events, ideas, and so forth. Therefore, emotions are an undependable aspect of carryover. One cannot build a carryover program around a client's feelings because feelings are always changing. The client may feel good about his progress in one moment, and then feel lousy about it the next. Emotions sway like a pendulum. Sometimes they sway just a little bit, and other times they swing dramatically from one extreme to another.

Clients will have more success in carryover if they learn to plow ahead despite changing emotions. In other words, the work of the SLP is to help the client carryover his new skills no matter how the emotions are felt from one moment to another. This means helping clients recognize how they are feeling about themselves, about their speech, and about the process of therapy. It also means helping the client take advantage of good feelings, and to rise above negative feelings that may arise during treatment and elsewhere. Van Riper and Irwin (1958) talked about helping clients desensitize themselves to what they called *extraneous emotional noise*:

> *"Every therapist knows that when the case is highly disturbed, embarrassed, or upset, the retraining goes slowly, the old errors tend to return to their old position of dominance. [The therapist] seeks therefore to create conditions so that such emotional noise will not interfere. But there is also need for therapy that will help the case to operate his new controls of articulation even in the presence of such disturbing influences"* (Van Riper and Irwin, 1958, p. 159).

Repressed Distress

Some clients do not generalize their new articulation skills outside of the therapy room because they hold themselves in check due to pent-up emotional distress related to the speech error. Release from distress can pave the way for carryover. Speech-language pathologists often must ask clients why they do not want to attend therapy, or why they are not trying these things outside of therapy. Sometimes I simply say, "You don't really seem to want to be here. What's going on with that?"

I am reminded here of an eleven-year-old boy who had bottled up shame about his frontal lisp. The emotional block seemed to have stemmed from severe criticism of his error by his mother. I do not know whether the parent actually was very harsh, or if this boy was just very sensitive, but he was fearful of change either way because of his repressed shame. The boy was cooperative in therapy, and was able to practice sounds and words with me, but he would not talk to me otherwise. He was holding something back. No spontaneous dialogue occurred, and I was beginning to wonder how to reach him because I knew that carryover would be in jeopardy if we did not move into conversation.

After a few weeks I took a chance and simply asked him straight out why he did not want to talk about anything, and he blurted out something about his mom being so mean and making him come to speech. Tears began to flow, and suddenly he stood up, declared he had to go to the bathroom, and ran out of the room. I think he left to cry because when he came back, he was composed, but his eyes were puffy and red. I did not ask him what had just happened because he started talking right away. I think he faced his fear, cried over it, and moved ahead in just those brief few minutes. This simple release of his pent-up emotion allowed him to move beyond single-words into dialogue. That was the day I realized that our methods sometimes have to reach into the psychological realm. In three decades of therapy I have encountered this type of problem in only a handful of clients, but releasing the block seemed to be a key to carryover for them: "We must always take into account the presence of emotional factors which might prevent the person from facing his speech defect" (Van Riper, 1947, p. 29).

Responding to New Feelings

Many clients encounter uncomfortable feelings during carryover, and responding well to them can be an important element for successful change. Allowing a client to express his feelings about speech change builds a bridge between therapy activities and the feelings the client encounters during the carryover process. The expression of feelings about speech work is as valuable in carryover as the speech production work itself. An emotional connection takes our therapy well beyond the simple process of practicing speech. It is a heart-to-heart connection that aids the carryover process. We have no research on this, of course.

Faber and Mazlish (1980) recommended five basic methods adults can use to help children express difficult feelings that arise during changing events. This simple book contains the material I used to learn how to deal with emotions expressed by my clients and my own children as well. The techniques they discussed are: *Listening, Acknowledging, Naming, Fantasizing*, and *Expressing*.

- LISTENING: Listen to a client express his feelings about his changing speech. Stop what you are doing, ignore the activity at hand, look the client in the eye, and simply pay attention to what he is saying. Overt signs of listening like this allow children to believe we are listening to them. Changing speech habits is not just an intellectual pursuit.

Speech-language pathologists must allow time for clients to express their feelings and observations so that the feeling connection is made. This doesn't have to happen in every session, but it should occur every once in a while.

- ACKNOWLEDGING: Acknowledge a client's expressed feelings of change with a simple word or comment. For example, a client who has been in therapy a while suddenly may blurt out, "I am sick of working on this!" We can acknowledge his feelings by making a simple comment like, "Oh, my gosh." Acknowledging a client's feelings with a few simple words reassures him by letting him know that it is all right to feel this way. Many of us would prefer to give advice in response to such comments. We want to say, "Now if you just stay with therapy and do your homework every week, you could get this over with..." But the client does not want this type of advice at this point, and he probably already knows it anyway. The client is just looking to express his emotion, and a simple acknowledgement lets him do so. Simple acknowledgements of the client's expressed feelings build trust. Our acknowledgements encourage a client to express an emotion and then let go of it so the work can continue.
- NAMING: Labeling an emotion encourages discussion about it. Clients sometimes express bad feelings about speech, for example, "My brother thinks going to speech is stupid." It is tempting for us to say something to cover up the emotion. We might say, "Don't feel bad... It'll be okay." But a cover-up remark like that denies the client's feelings. Instead Faber and Mazlish recommended that we name the emotion by saying, for example, "That must feel *awful*." Naming the emotion gives a reality to it and makes it something the two of you can observe and discuss. Naming the feeling connects the work being done in the treatment room in an emotional way to the rest of the client's life.
- FANTASIZING: Most adults tend to use logic in response to a client's feelings, and we try to explain their feelings away with reason. But reasoned responses distance us from our clients. For example, a client who is working on R may lament, "I wish I could live in Japan. They don't have to say R in Japan." Logic would cause us to respond with reason by saying, for example, "Now you know that you're not going to be able to move to Japan..." Logic like this stifles emotional expression, and it is the emotional expression that we are trying to allow in order to foster carryover. Instead of using logic, we can use fantasy to help the client realize how much we understand what he is going through. We might say, "Yes, that would be perfect! Then you wouldn't have to remember to say R at all. I wonder how much an airline ticket to Japan would cost?" Take a moment to dream up the cost of an airline ticket to Japan. Let the client fantasize about what it would feel like not to have this burden, and then get back to work. Encouraging a client's imagination sets him free because he begins to trust that you will not shame him for these thoughts. The work of carryover then becomes integral to his imaginative life.
- EXPRESS YOUR OWN FEELINGS: Another way to get a client to express his own feelings about carryover is to express your own feelings about it. For example, make a purposeful error and then say with a little misery, "I hate it when I make mistakes like that. I know how to do it. I should be able to do it right all the time." Our expression of our own feelings allows clients to open up about their feeling, and this builds rapport and commitment to the process of carryover.

Ten Things to Avoid When Children Express New Feelings

Faber and Mazlish also advised parents to avoid ten things when children express newfound emotions during any process of change. These ideas can be applied to the carryover process:

1. Don't ask the client why he is feeling the way he does. That only adds to his problem.
2. Don't say you agree with the feeling. Just acknowledge it.
3. Don't say that you understand what the child is feeling. The child will not believe you.
4. Don't take an insult personally. State that the insult hurt your feelings, but move past it quickly.
5. Don't forget to set limits on behavior when feelings are expressed. For example, it's okay for the client to say, "That makes me mad." But it is not okay for him to throw furniture around when he says it.
6. Don't give advice when accepting feelings. That deprives the client the ability simply to feel his feeling.
7. Don't repeat the child's exact words back to him. It will upset him further.
8. Don't forget that some clients will prefer to stay quiet when they are upset, but they may be able to talk about it later.
9. Don't respond with more intensity than the client originally expressed. Don't make the feelings bigger than they are.
10. Don't repeat ugly names back to the client as you are mirroring his feelings.

Fear of Someone Noticing the Change

Carryover fails in some clients because they would rather keep an error that they think no one notices. They are afraid to change because they fear that the change itself will make people think there is something wrong with them. This is quite a dilemma for these clients. They want to change for the purpose of change, but they don't want to change because they don't want anyone to notice the change. I employ two interconnected strategies when this situation arises. I tell my clients that I know a secret that will help them, and I tell them that there is a simple way to test it. My secret is that very few people—probably no one—will notice the change they make in their speech. Then I help the client identify one person with whom they can test out this secret.

Help the client find one person with whom he can test this theory. This must be a person who feels safe to the client, not someone we pick for him. I let my clients have free reign in this selection, and I am often amused at their choices. This person probably will not be a parent, sibling, or best friend. In fact, people close to the client may be the last choice. Many clients seem to select a person connected to their life in a small way, like the cafeteria lady, the school custodian, the bus driver, or the person behind the counter at McDonald's. One boy chose his dog. Once the conversational partner is chosen, we select something to say to them, and we discuss the logistics. Then the client reports back to me in the next session.

My experience is that most clients realize the secret is true—that other people don't even notice the change they have made. This gives the client confidence to try another person. Soon the client realizes that carrying over the new skill to conversations with everyone else is not so scary after all. This can be the moment of carryover breakthrough for clients who are plagued by this fear of being noticed. The dialogue box in Table 3 provides an example of this. It is an interaction between a teenage client and an SLP. Read the dialogue left-to-right and line-by-line from top to bottom to see how the therapist helps the client deal with his fear that someone will notice that he is correcting his error.

Table 3 – Client in R Therapy

Client	Therapist
…and then I realized that I had to say helicopter, and man…	What?
Oh, man. That R was in there. I was freaking.	Oh, yea… *Helicopter* has that huge R at the end. What did you do?
Well, I had to say it. My report was all about helicopters.	And you didn't think of it ahead of time?
No, I knew helicopter had an R, but I completely forgot that I had to read it in front of the whole class.	You had to read it in front of the entire class?
Yea.	Yikes…
Yea, so all of a sudden I was freaking out.	That's a bad feeling.
Yea it is. Totally freaking. I didn't want to go up there. But I had to read it…	Did you do any of the sounds wrong?
Yea… About half.	You did half of them wrong?
Ummm… Yea, about half.	Well that's good.
That's good?	Yes. Because that means that you did half of them right!
Oh yea…	Half is excellent. Congratulations.
I didn't think I did so good.	If you did half correctly, you did perfectly.
Really?	Yes. Because, remember three months ago, you couldn't do any of the words correctly.

continued on page 100

Client	Therapist
Right...	So half is outstanding.
Yea. It is good, isn't it?	And what happened? Did anybody say anything?
No.	You mean they didn't even notice?
No. I don't think anyone even noticed.	Hmmm...That's probably right. No one even noticed.
Yea.	That's good.
Huh?	That's good because then it doesn't matter if you try to do it the new way.
Oh, yea.	Right?
What?	When you do it right, no one hardly notices that anything is different. Remember, that's the secret.
What's that secret again?	Very few people will notice when you change the sound and make it correctly.
Oh, yea...	Excellent.

Personality Domains

A client's personality plays into the selection of carryover techniques. *Personality* is "the combination of characteristics or qualities that form an individual's distinctive character" (Jewell and Abate, 2001, p. 1276). One school of thought (e.g., Eysenck, 1990) has been to organize people into to five basic personality domains: *Openness, Consciousness, Extroversion, Agreeableness,* and *Neuroticism.* These five personality types can help us form a framework in decision-making about the types of carryover techniques one might employ with specific clients. Although the SLP typically is not qualified to make a diagnosis of personality, most of us know people fairly well and can make excellent observations of behavior. Therefore we can make general decisions about our clients' personalities in order to design useful carryover techniques for each one. We can assume that there is overlap of these domains.

1. OPENNESS: Some clients are open to new experiences. They love art, have no fear of emotional expression, are adventurous, have deeply rooted intellectual curiosity, tend

to prefer a variety of experiences, and are sensitive to beauty. These clients might be more apt to develop carryover skills when a variety of methods are employed. Use painting, drawing, creative writing, and other expression oriented projects for carryover. Also allow these clients to discuss how they feel about the therapy process. Drillwork may be much too boring for these clients as they will see no purpose in it unless it is tied to their intellectual curiosity or creative drive.

2. CONSCIOUSNESS: Some clients are efficient, organized, self-disciplined, dutiful, and achievement oriented. They like to have a plan of action. These clients might be more apt to develop carryover skills when very specific tasks are assigned, when drill is included, when strict behavior management routines are utilized, and when therapists monitor progress carefully. These clients will not be offended by close scrutiny of homework assignments. In fact, they will love your detailed assistance and will view it as instructive. They will seek your approval and will appreciate meaningful rewards.
3. EXTROVERSION: Some clients are outgoing, energetic, urgent, expressive of positive emotions, and have a tendency to seek the company of others. They like to say, "Yes!" They also like to talk and draw attention to themselves. Carryover activities that involve being out in the world will be the most fun for them. These clients can be wonderful to send into classrooms to do speech improvement lessons with younger children because they will enjoy explaining their own speech skills to others. In the one-on-one therapy setting, these clients may simply want to talk about themselves. In the small group, these clients may be the ones around whom the others flock. Immediate gratification will go far in their carryover program.
4. AGREEABLENESS: Some clients are friendly, compassionate, and cooperative. They are generous and seek social harmony. They will compromise easily and will want to please the therapist and all others involved in the process. They believe in the essential goodness of people. Carryover techniques that may be the most beneficial to these clients may involve group work, cooperative learning experiences, and community projects. Projects involving teaching or nurturing small children, tending animals, or caring for the environment may be attractive as carryover assignments. These clients will do almost any homework assignment because that is the nice thing to do. They will work toward carryover if you tell them it is important.
5. NEUROTICISM: Some clients are sensitive, nervous, and insecure. They have a tendency to experience negative emotions such as anxiety, anger, and depression. They feel vulnerable and are reactive. They get in bad moods. These clients may be very wary of their own ability to succeed in therapy, and they may feel very afraid to try their new skills with others outside of the therapy room. They may agree to a carryover assignment, but then fail to act because they didn't feel right about the assignment when it came time to do it. Enlisting the client's own ideas about how to achieve carryover probably will be the best attack. Allow these clients time to express their fear, and redirect their negative self-talk. Draw clear lines between acceptable and unacceptable speech. These clients may work harder when their self-image is boosted.

Ego-Building Statements

Making ego-building comments to a client is not considered a valid aspect of behavior modification so we omitted it from that chapter. But building up the ego should be discussed here because it is an effective tool in all aspects of speech training, especially in the carryover process. Whereas positive and negative reinforcement are used to give feedback about specific behaviors, ego-building comments are made to stimulate the client to believe in himself and his ability to change. This is a type of brainwashing that indoctrinates a client into believing in himself. It helps him begin to believe that he is a good person, that he is smart, that he is determined, and that he can be successful in this work.

Each speech-language pathologist will approach this in his or her own way. I prefer to build my clients up with positive statements about who they are, what they are accomplishing, and how quickly they are progressing. I have never found a client who did not like this when used in moderation. Parents also like to hear us speak well of their children, and ego-building comments made about the child can be a way to compliment parents too. Here are a few examples:

- "Wow. You are doing so great today. I did not realize how quickly you could learn this."
- "Did you know that most kids couldn't do that the first day of speech? It's true. That is really hard to do. But you managed it just fine. You are going to do great here."
- "You guys are amazing! I was sure you all were going to mess that up today, but you didn't. I am impressed. How old are guys? … Only eleven? Really? I was thinking that you were twelve already. All three of you are very mature for sixth graders."
- "Mary worked really hard today. I am happy you brought her to me. I really like working with her."
- "Don't worry about Daniel. He is so smart he is going to figure this out in no time."

Ego-building comments push a client toward carryover because they stimulate the client's good feelings about himself and about the process of change. The client discovers that thinking about speech work makes him feel good, and he will want to re-create these feelings outside of therapy. The client learns to use his process of speech change to regulate his feel-good brain chemistry, and he will begin to use his good speech more often as a result. Ego-building statements are used every so often in a program built on a solid foundation of good behavior management.

Reverse Psychology

The concept of *reverse psychology* can be used as a very effective method of bringing conscious control over speech skills in the process of building carryover. Reverse psychology is the process of telling a person to do the opposite of what you really want him to do. It is a basic psychological concept. To motivate carryover one might say, "I hope you are not trying to say these sounds with anyone else," or, "I don't think you will ever remember this when you are not with me!"

Reverse psychology is an especially good method for clients whose personalities or stage of development motivate them always to do the opposite of what they are told. This is like working with a two-year-old whose cognitive level forces him to balk whenever he is told what to do. I have used reverse psychology successfully in this way with many different types of clients, including those with whom I am trying to motivate carryover. Reverse psychology works for a certain time period until the client catches on. But even after discovery, reverse psychology can continue to be used if done in a humorous and teasing way. Consider the therapist who dramatically says, "No! No! Please don't use your new sound with anyone else! That would be terrible! Then they will find out what we are doing in here!" Children love to play with these ideas as they learn to manipulate these psychological constructs: "Some children work best if you bet they can't do something. They take great delight in proving you wrong. Their only demand is that you be dramatically surprised" (Bosley, 1981, p. 26).

Self-Talk

The psychological term *self-talk* has relevance to carryover. Self-talk is the running dialogue that each of us has about who we are. It is part of our self-esteem. Some of this self-talk is positive and some is negative. The speech-language pathologist's job is to help clients change any self-talk that interferes with carryover. We must re-iterate that speech-language pathologists are not psychologists, but there are certain methods for changing self-talk that can be found today in self-help books and magazines, and in on-line advice blogs. Anyone can employ these methods in their personal life, and speech-language pathologists can employ them to promote carryover in their articulation clients. Here are some examples:

- AWARENESS: Help the client realize that he is rehearsing negative ideas about his speech. For example, the client may say, "I can't do it." Tell him, "Yes you can." Teach the story of *The Little Engine That Could.*
- HALT THE PROCESS: Teach the client to stop the thought process that is interfering with carryover. When he begins to belittle his skill, say, "Don't go there. Don't tell yourself that."
- RE-WORDING: Teach the client to change negative statements into positive ones. Change the statement, "I don't know how to do this," to, "I am figuring out how to do this."
- EXPECTATIONS: Teach the client to change his use of *should* to *want*. For example, change, "I should say my sound correctly all the time," to, "I want to say my sound correctly all the time." This type of change takes the pressure off and helps the client realize that he has a choice in the matter.
- EXTREME THINKING: Teach the client to limit extreme thinking. Change, "I will never fix this," to, "I am learning how to fix this." This type of change brings reality into focus.
- JUMPING TO CONCLUSIONS: Teach the client to stop jumping to conclusions about his speech. Change, "I only have one friend because I can't say R," to, "I have a friend who plays with me every day even though I am still learning R." This type of change can help to eliminate degrading ideas that are interfering with carryover.
- JOURNAL WRITING: Journal writing has long been recognized as a way to identify hidden feelings and negative self-talk. It can be used with older clients to help them recognize the limitations they are placing upon themselves.

Stress at Home

Some of our clients cannot carry their speech work home because the home is an unsettled place. Serious problems like drug or alcohol abuse may preclude any possibility of carryover homework. Less threatening problems like poor parental management or general chaos also can interfere with home activities. Even common problems like busy schedules or sibling rivalry can interfere with carryover. Some clients even must be dismissed from therapy until the home life improves. I am reminded here of a seven-year-old boy with an R and L distortion. He was quite stimulable during his evaluation, but the parents were in the middle of a divorce. I could not see any good coming of therapy at that time. Therapy was initiated two years later after the home life settled down.

Speech-language pathologists usually cannot fix these types of problems, but we can be a willing listener, and we can teach our clients a little bit about coping under such circumstances. Of course it is the speech-language pathologist's duty to report home life infractions if they are serious, but often we simply have to teach clients to ignore what is happening at home and to focus on what they can accomplish with us in therapy. We help our clients understand that they can be all they want to be despite the things that are happening around them.

Teasing

Bad feelings can arise when clients are teased about their speech, and a client's immature reaction to teasing can stifle carryover. I have always followed my mother's advice when it comes to helping my clients swallow this bitter pill. I teach them to rise above teasing. I tell my clients that teasing is very bad behavior and that they are better than the child who is resorting to teasing. I teach them that they do not have to pay attention to the child or his taunts, and that they should feel sorry for the other child because he or she does not understand this. I inform my clients that they are doing very well, that they should not worry about what others think or say, and that they should plow through to victory despite what anyone else thinks about what they are doing. I teach my clients the old rhyme adults used to teach all children:

> *Sticks and stones*
> *May break my bones*
> *But words can never hurt me!*

Such simple advice seems to be missing in the world today. We can accomplish so much when we do what is best and ignore the naysayers! I teach my clients not to let other people dictate who they are or what they are becoming. I teach them to be strong in the face of adversity. I teach them that they will feel bad periodically when others tease them, but so what? I teach them to let go of the bad feeling and move on. I teach them that if they let others control them they will stay in therapy for the rest of their lives. Most clients respond quite well to encouragement such as this.

CAVEAT: Clients who cannot seem to adopt a positive attitude because they are chronically down or depressed should be referred for psychological evaluation. Also, teasing that has become bullying, psychological abuse, or physical harm should be reported immediately.

Varying the Emotional Background

Van Riper and Irwin (1958) wrote that some clients resort to old familiar and incorrect patterns of speech when highly charged, embarrassed, or upset. They suggested that carryover would not reach completion until these clients could produce their new sounds under conditions of varying emotional stress. They suggested that we introduce various emotions in therapy so the client can learn to hold true to his new production as his emotions change.

> *"Emotion is like static on the radio — it interferes with the reception of messages ... Therefore, as our final task of therapy, we have to teach the case to use his new sounds under conditions of emotion"* (Van Riper and Irwin, 1958, p. 118).

Despite this early admonition, the process of working with emotional variations seems to have been dropped from modern textbooks on articulation and phonology. This may have begun in the 1980's when Polson's (1980) study indicated that speech-language pathologists working in the public schools considered emotional variations to be one of the least important of twelve factors in the carryover process. The view reflected in textbooks since then seems to be that emotion is not an important factor in articulation therapy.

But my experience is that working on emotional variations is important for carryover with at least one type of client — the client who loses control when he is excited. Certain types of clients lose complete control of speech as soon as they get wound up, and carryover is almost always a big problem with them. Speech-language pathologists build excitement into therapy activities so that these clients can learn to maintain control as their enthusiasm builds. Even though we have no data to back up this claim, common sense dictates that certain clients must learn to say their targets no matter how interesting, amusing, or exciting an event may be. This should aid the carryover process for them.

Varying the emotional background can mean different things for different clients. A high functioning client who is working on a specific phoneme in words can be required to use his best level of performance while playing a fast and furious card game. The therapist might tell the client that she is going to try to get him to forget his sounds during the game. The game is purposefully challenging and contains dares and elements of sabotage to throw the client into a friendly tizzy. The client learns to control his speech as he gets worked up.

A younger child, or one with little expressive language, may need a different approach to varying the emotional setting. For example, a toddler may be able to say *bye-bye* to his mom when she leaves the room but be unable to produce the word while waving good-bye to a group of loud motorcycles roaring by the window. The child's SLP must help him do both.

Passions and Pursuits

Some clients are not interested in carryover because they have no awareness that speech improvement has any relevance to their passions and pursuits. In fact they may believe that speech work is interfering with their real interests. A client like that will have no reason to monitor his speech outside of the therapy room, and carryover will be nearly impossible. Self-monitoring for carryover is almost guaranteed, however, once we connect to their present interests. This connection of speech work to present life can be made through a discussion of the client's favorite activities. Using a client's favorite topics to promote carryover is discussed in many traditional articulation textbooks. It is a standard teaching method that has been applied to many teaching fields.

One of the best examples of this from my own experience is that of a 12-year-old boy named Clay who came to me to learn a correct R. Clay didn't like coming to speech, and he was extremely frustrated by his unsuccessful participation in therapy during years past. In addition, Clay liked to play lacrosse and he felt that our after school speech work was interfering with his focus on the sport. I knew nothing about lacrosse, having never even watched a game, so I stopped working on R-words and began to ask him about it. I then began to weave the topic of lacrosse into our speech work. Together Clay and I hunted down R-words while we engaged in a variety of activities with lacrosse as the topic:

- We drew sketchy pictures of the field, and named all the lines, goals, benches and so forth.
- We labeled the play positions and discussed some of the plays he knew.
- We talked about the name of his team, who came up with it, and what it meant.
- We listed the coaches. He talked about which coaches were great and which ones he wished would quit.
- We listed the players. He talked about the team members who played fair and those who didn't, who were the best, and so forth.
- We went to the website that one of the players' dads had created for the client's team, and we talked about the schedule posted there. We read the dates of the games, the opposing team names, and the match locations. We also read the rainy day policy and some of the rules of the game.
- We talked about the uniforms and equipment. Clay brought his uniform into therapy one day and this seemed very gratifying for him. He was quite proud of that uniform, having mowed lawns to help pay for it. This day may have been the key to carryover because Clay began to speak very rapidly and naturally about his uniform, and he was using correct R sounds.
- We made word lists about lacrosse that we organized by topic. We highlighted those words that contained his target sound, and we used those words as practice material for the rest of his treatment.
- We wrote a story about a boy who played lacrosse.

Clay blossomed during this six-week period. He marveled at how prevalent the R sound was in the vocabulary of lacrosse: "I can't believe how many R's there are!" What had been the drudgery of going to speech became a weekly thrill for him. He finally had found someone with whom he could discuss the game he loved so much, someone who would listen to his every word and respond accordingly. Focusing therapy on Clay's passion for lacrosse established my rapport with him beyond anything else I could have done. Our word lists became *his* word lists, and our speech work became completely functional for him. From that point forward conversation with Clay became easier, and I found he began to speak on any number of other subjects. This switch from my topics to his topic became the key to carryover for this boy, and he now had a solid reason to monitor his speech.

*

Chapter 8 Summary

Personality, Emotion, and Attitude in Carryover

- A client's desire to improve his speech is a powerful force in obtaining carryover.
- Good rapport between the therapist and client is necessary to build carryover skill.
- Therapists encourage clients to use new speech skills outside the speech room just as a coach might encourage a team to play well in the next game.
- Sometimes the best thing we can do for carryover is to take the pressure off.
- Clients have more success in carryover if they learn to plow ahead despite changing emotions.
- Release of pent-up emotional distress can pave the way for carryover.
- Allowing clients to express their feelings about speech change builds a bridge between therapy and everyday life.
- Carryover fails in some clients because they would rather keep an error that they think no one notices.
- A client's personality plays into the selection of carryover techniques.
- Ego-building comments are made to stimulate the client to believe in himself and his ability to change.
- Reverse psychology is an especially good method of carryover for clients whose personalities or stage of development motivate them to do the opposite of what they are told.
- Speech-language pathologists help clients change any self-talk that interferes with carryover.
- Speech-language pathologists usually cannot fix big problems that interfere with carryover at home, but we can be a willing listener, and we can teach our clients a little bit about coping under such circumstances.
- Therapists teach clients how to plow through to victory despite the naysayers.
- Speech-language pathologists build excitement into therapy activities so that clients can learn to maintain control as enthusiasm builds.
- Self-monitoring for carryover is almost guaranteed once we connect the speech work to a client's passions and pursuits.

Chapter 9

Games and Activities to Promote Carryover

"This final stage of therapy must not be left to chance."

– Marvin Hanson, 1983

Games and activities are the nuts and bolts of daily therapy. Games and activities can be included from the first day of therapy, and they can be used as a backdrop for practicing all manner of speech skills. These are the activities that make in-room speech work more like the speech children use outside of the therapy room. Games and other activities create a bridge from the rehearsal of words to the production of spontaneous conversation. A child who can control his speech while getting caught up in the excitement of games and activities is learning how to be in command of his speech in unstructured situations. This is the ultimate skill he needs for success in carryover.

Some of the games and activities of this final chapter are very cognitive in nature, and they make children think harder for carryover. Other ideas are playful and fun, and they lighten up the heavy load that speech correction can be at times. The competitive games contained herein are useful because they start out slowly and gain speed and energy within the session, thus reinforcing the notion that increasing and not decreasing speed of production is that which ultimately facilitates carryover. Some of these ideas help develop conscious control in the classroom or at home. Most importantly, many of these activities stimulate humor. Children who can hold their speech together while giggling and laughing may have reached the pinnacle of carryover success.

Common sense, working theories, creative drive, and natural teaching ability are behind all of the ideas presented in this chapter. None have undergone systematic research as far as I know. Why would they need to be? These are the types of activities about which Charles Van Riper and John Irwin said, "There are no doubt almost as many ways of carrying out these basic principles as there are clinicians" (Van Riper and Irwin, 1958, p. 118). Some of these ideas come from old textbooks on articulation therapy and others are old stand-bys of unknown origin. Some of these ideas stem from my own clinical experience. Many of these ideas were submitted by other speech-language pathologists.

My original intention was to divide the ideas of this chapter into four groups — therapy activities, classroom activities, home activities, and car activities. Then I realized that a great number of these ideas could be used in any setting if only slight modifications were made. Therefore these games and activities simply are presented in alphabetical order with no organization or hierarchy implied. These activities should be done in conjunction with all the ideas presented in our earlier chapters. Please keep in mind that these ideas are designed to help clients with carryover. None are intended to teach clients how to produce their phonemes correctly in the first place.

Bingo Adaptations

Many therapists use adaptations of the game of Bingo in speech. Gailyn Walsh Ryan uses a form of Bingo for carryover. She makes a card with a bingo-like grid using a spread sheet. Then she talks to the client about the things he does outside of school — such as eating dinner, riding in the car, playing outside, spending time in the family room, and so forth. She types the name of one activity in each square of the card. She adds instructions for parents on the card. The instructions tell parents to initial each square that represents when the child has spoken correctly for fifteen minutes in that setting. When the child receives initials in a horizontal, vertical, or diagonal line, he returns the card to speech for a prize.

Bird Watching

Ellen Obrock developed a bird-watching activity for carryover. She writes, "The kids love it and it's motivating. Who doesn't love looking at birds? The names of the birds always have an R, S or L. It costs nothing [and] it can become a lifelong hobby." Ellen reported several different things clients could do to promote carryover with their bird-watching activity. She reminds us that this type of activity can be used with any topic, not just birds. The important thing is to use a subject that can wow others. These are the types of things they do:

- Practice the names of the birds that visit the client's yard.
- Describe the various attributes of the birds.
- Impress family members by telling them the bird names: "Hey, that's a Red-headed Woodpecker!"
- Make a scrapbook about birds.
- Build a bird feeder.
- Learn to make birdcalls.
- Use birds as a show-and-tell activity.
- Create a bulletin board about birds with magazine and Internet pictures.
- Learn some advanced words related to birds, e.g., *ornithology*.

Board Games and Card Games

Many therapists submitted idea for the use of individual board or card games. From simple board games like *Chutes and Ladders* to card games like *War*, board and card games seem to be some of the most common ideas for carryover. There are too many board and card games to discuss each one individually here. The basic idea is twofold: (1) Take any game and highlight the speech targets within the game, or (2) Take any game and modify it so that speech targets can be included. We can modify any game to include more target phonemes by changing the name of game pieces, cards, or procedures. For example, the *Go to Jail* card in the game of *Monopoly* can be changed to a different name depending upon what phoneme is being targeted for carryover. Here are a few examples:

- R — *Run to the Secure Prison Right Now*
- S — *Skedaddle to the Secure Safety Cell Instantly*
- Sh — *Shuttle to the Shameful Shack with the Sheriff*
- Ch — *Hitch a Choo-choo to the Chump Room*
- F — *Fly to the Felony Fort Fast*
- L — *Leap to the Unlucky Losers Locked Cell*
- Th — *Throw the Thieving Thieves into the Theft Theater*

Body Outlines

Barbara Miller uses the old body tracing activity for carryover with young children. Children lie down on a piece of large butcher paper, and an outline is made around the whole body from head to toe. The picture is rolled up and sent home for the kids to decorate. Together with their family they have to come up with words that contain their sounds, for example, *head, heart, hip*, and *hands* for H. They also come up with words to describe broader ideas having to do with the body parts, for example, *headache*, *hold a hammer*, or *have happy feelings*.

Calendars

Many therapists use calendars for carryover. Give the client a photocopied calendar to take home. Have the child bring it back at the end of the month in order to get a reward. The client will use the calendar in a prescribed way. For example:

- Challenge the child to say his sound every day. Have him place a stamp, sticker, or star on each day he remembers.
- Give the client a calendar on which you have written one target word for each day. Write the words down together. Challenge the child to use each word in conversation three times on the day it is posted. Have him mark the days he completes the task.
- Give the client a blank calendar for him to post words he hears during each day. The task is for the client to listen to others speak, to listen for target words, and to write these down on the calendar day. When the client returns the calendar, he will tell the therapist about the individual postings — who said them, what the circumstances were, and so forth.
- Kelly Davis gives her students a calendar to do over the summer break. On each day is posted something the children can do to promote carryover. Parents sign the calendars, or initial each day's activity. Kelly collects these calendars when the children return in the fall, and she rewards them for their summer work. As examples, day squares might say:

- Name five flowers with your sound.
- How many ice cream flavors have your sound?
- Talk about how a butterfly and an airplane are the same and different using your sound.
- What do you see at a pool that has your sound?
- What do you do on the Fourth of July that has your sound?
- What do you like about not being in school that has your sound?

Card / Magic Tricks

Sherri Hole suggests that therapists who know how to do a few simple card or magic tricks can teach clients to do them with their deck of speech cards. Sherri reports that those of us who do not know any of these tricks can find them on the Internet by searching under *free easy magic tricks*. I have never used this idea in therapy because I simply never thought of it. But this is an excellent idea because children love card and magic tricks! Teach the client to do a trick or two, and then have him put on a little show for others. Have him teach his parents and other children how to do the tricks, too.

Catch 'em While They're Good

Lois B. Cook trains her clients' parents for carryover by leading them in an activity she calls *Catch 'em While They're Good.* Early in therapy, and months before carryover begins, Lois works with parents to teach them how to use positive reinforcement to promote good behavior of all kinds. The parents first learn how to say positive things to one another. In essence, they learn how to notice the little things their spouse does around the house, and to say, "I love how you ____." For example, "I love how you picked up the mail on the way in." Training mothers and fathers in this way assures Lois that they will be able to use positive reinforcement during their student's carryover activities when the time comes. This is such an excellent idea for carryover training. I am sure Lois is helping a few marriages along the way with this idea as well.

Catcher Game

Nicole Spruill designed a simple game called *The Catcher* to stimulate the retention of sounds or syllables in conversation. The client and therapist take turns talking extemporaneously about a toy, picture, or object. The speaker speaks, and the listener listens. If the listener hears the speaker delete a sound or syllable, then she pretends to catch the error in a real or imaginary hat. A caught sound or syllable scores a point for the catcher. The players alternate turns until one reaches a predetermined winning score. I like this game because it requires no preparation, because it would work with individuals and groups, and because a therapist could initiate a turn or two of this game anywhere outside of the therapy session simply by using her fist to grab the escaping sounds. Children also could play it with each other in the car or elsewhere. The game also could be played with more imaginary play, like pretending the escaping sounds and syllables were butterflies and the listener was using a net to catch them.

Collages

The process of constructing collages is very conducive to the stimulation of spontaneous speech around specific speech targets. The classic way to do this is to use pictures, photographs, and words cut from magazines. Today children can bring in pictures they have printed off the Internet too. Have the children find pictures and words that contain their sounds. Glue them on paper to make a two-dimensional collage, or glue them to objects to make three-dimensional art. For example, decorate a shoebox to hold keepsakes. Almost any object can be used, just make sure to use the appropriate type of glue for each. Use the construction time to stimulate spontaneous conversation about the project, or use it as a platform to discuss any number of subjects.

Chips

Many therapists wrote that they use plastic poker chips in numerous ways during conversations in therapy. Chips are given to and taken away from clients based on performance, and rewards are offered for the one with the most at the end of the session. Chips are gathered in pockets, pails, boxes, bowls, or bags. These general procedures are employed:

- The child starts with no chips. He earns a chip for every correct sound he makes in the conversation.
- The child receives a certain number of chips at the beginning of the session. He relinquishes one chip every time he makes and error in conversation.
- Children in a group each get a certain number of chips. They give and take chips from one another when they say sounds correctly and when they catch each other making sounds incorrectly.

Classroom Visits

Mary Jane Thomas has a simple yet very effective way to induce carryover in her students. She rearranges her schedule so she can visit their classrooms during special events. She does this so she can hear their spontaneous speech. For example, she visits the kindergarten during *Bring and Tell* (*Show and Tell*) and she visits the first and second graders during *Star of the Week*. She does not interact with the students during this time. She just listens. Then she comments on their speech the next time she sees them in the therapy setting.

Clicker Counter / Tally Counter Activities

Susan Freiman Ross has her clients play a clicker counter game for home carryover. A client and his parent have daily conversations while each holds a clicker counter. Whenever one of them says a word containing the target sound correctly, he or she gets to click their counter. If they misarticulate, or if they miss a click, the other person gets to capture the word by clicking. A goal is set at perhaps 100 clicks. Whoever achieves the designated number of clicks first is the winner. Susan says she loves this game because the movement and sound of clicking reinforces the correct sound, and because the activity promotes both production and auditory discrimination.

Susan Cohn uses clickers to count correct productions, and then has clients color in dots on a picture of a leopard after they have reached a certain number of clicks. The leopard pictures are posted with the kids' names inside her therapy room, and the children love to check to see who is getting the most dots. As the children get better, and the number of correct productions and clicks increase in conversation, she then begins to count the number of errors made by using a different noisemaker. For example, she may use a frog squeaky toy for error productons. Now she clicks for correct productions and squeaks for incorrect ones. When the frog squeaks, she places a small plastic coin in a *Boo-boo Basket*. At the end of the session, they count the number of boo-boos, and subtract that number from the correct productions noted on the clicker counter. The child gets to color in the final or net number on the picture.

Clothespins in a Bottle

Dropping clothespins into a bottle is a game that can be used for carryover. The game goes way back; I remember playing it as a five-year-old child at a birthday party for one of my neighbors in 1958, and I am sure my mother even played the game back in the 1930's. I found the game mentioned in a few speech texts published before 1960. People don't use clothespins much any more, but they still can be purchased in grocery, drug, and variety stores. Use the type that pinches closed so the clothespins can be attached to the client's cards.

Place a wide-mouthed bottle or jar on the floor — mayonnaise jars work well. The child's job is to select a card, name it, remove the clothespin, and then drop the clothespin into the jar. Have the children stand behind the jar, or have them kneel on a chair next to the jar, and drop the clothespin in from eye level. This is a simple game that can be used at any level of therapy. But getting the pin into the bottle is not as easy as it seems, and the difficulty causes much conversation about the task. Talk about which pins went in the jar during and after the game: "I got book in but I couldn't do bike or bake!" Keep score, and compare scores over time. Write a summary paragraph about how well the children did to remember and share with others. The children should get better at dropping the pins in as the term of therapy progresses.

Coins

Some therapists use real coins as an incentive for working on carryover in the therapy room or at home. For example, Anne Venables Eigner has parents sit at a table across from the child and place a row of coins on the table between them. The coins are given to the child and he can keep them as long as he uses good speech. A cup of tea, a photo album, or another prop sets the stage. The parent and child engage in conversation on any topic. As they talk, the parent takes one coin away every time she hears the child make an error, and she takes two away if she has to help the child correct himself. Anne find that this activity encourages students to develop sharper self-monitoring skills.

Coupon Holders

Denise Davis submitted a very nice idea for sending speech work home for carryover. She uses coupon holders, you know, the type that you use to sort and carry coupons to the grocery store. When a child can say a word correctly in therapy, she makes a photocopy of the card to send home. The child and parent color and cut out the picture at home, and they put it in the coupon holder. They talk about the picture and the process throughout. These coupon holders with the cards inside go back and forth from home and school. This seems like a very nice and neat way to keep in touch with the parents regularly.

Dice and Spinners

Dice are used in any number of games, and children should be required to call out the numbers in order to stimulate their spontaneous production. Individual die carry the numbers 1–6 with their consonants — W, N, T, Th, Thr, F, R, V, S and K. When two dice are thrown, new numbers are added — 7, 8, 9, 10, 11, 12. Even more numbers arise when three dice are thrown, and so forth. Some dice are made with alphabet letters, and these can be used as well. Simply roll the dice and have the children call out the letters. Spinning wheels with letters, numbers, or colors afford the same type of practice.

Dictionaries and Other Books About Words

I have always relied on dictionaries to provide me with a plethora of reading and discussion material for speech practice at the carryover level. I keep dictionaries of all types and levels in my therapy room, from picture dictionaries designed for preschoolers, to the authorized *New Oxford American Dictionary* (Jewell and Abate, 2001). A discussion of words, their pronunciation, their history and origin, and their multiple definitions makes for a near perfect speech therapy activity to get adolescents interested in words and sounds. I also use rhyming dictionaries and encyclopedias for this purpose. The classic reference called *40,000 Selected Words: Organized by Letter, Sound, and Syllable* (Blockcolsky, Frazer, and Frazer, 1987) is another interesting book that adolescents love to explore. Dictionaries for young children often contain sentences with the word instead of a definition of the word. Very inexpensive dictionaries and encyclopedias can be found at used bookstores and library closeouts. Often they are found in the box of free toys at garage sales.

Dolls

Do not overlook the value of dolls, especially Barbie dolls, when working on carryover. Doll play generates much spontaneous speech as children imagine life as a parent (while playing with baby dolls) or as an independent adult (while playing with Barbie and Ken dolls). Even older children who are beyond doll play like to play with dolls periodically as they reminisce about how they "used to play with dolls." I have always kept various collections of dolls, doll clothes, dollhouses, doll furniture, and doll vehicles for spontaneous production work with all sorts of clients.

Felt Boards

Kim Metzgar reminds us that felt boards are an excellent way to stimulate spontaneous speech. Therapists always used to make their own felt boards and shapes, but today there are felt board sets of colors, numbers, letters, animals, vehicles, holidays, and so forth. There are sets that portray classic children's stories like *Goldie Locks and the Three Bears*. Some speech cards can have felt or Velcro glued on the back for use with a felt board. Felt is rather inexpensive to purchase at a craft or sewing store, and children who can handle a rather sharp pair of good sewing scissors can make their own shapes. Felt board play makes an excellent way to practice and use target words spontaneously as the scene unfolds.

Field Trips

I have used field trips with selected clients for carryover. I have taken clients to shopping malls, movie theaters, museums, pet stores, restaurants, and ice cream parlors. I have taken them on carousel and ferry boat rides. I took one to the top of the Space Needle in Seattle. I invited another to spend the day with me at my home so he could play with my daughters and my dogs. I have taken clients with me to purchase groceries for my therapy room, and I have taken them to local playgrounds and on walks around the neighborhood. Any place can be a field trip. Plan it out ahead of time and talk about it afterwards. Use the client's speech words throughout. Make sure to obtain written parent permission in advance.

Five-Minute Therapy Homework

As was mentioned earlier, some therapists who work in the schools prefer to see students several times per week for five minutes at a time. Jane Moerman has a specific plan when she operates this way that she finds to be an excellent way to include parents in the carryover process. During the five-minute therapy session, the children imitate or spontaneously produce prepared lists of words, phrases, or sentences. Jane writes down the utterances the client says incorrectly on a strip of paper that she sends home with the student. The students are to practice these words with their parents in the evening. The parents sign the slip, and the children return it the next session. Jane finds that this activity helps parents come to a better understand of what their child is learning in speech, and it helps them begin to realize that it only takes five minutes of an evening to work on it. Jane's slip of paper contains a place to write the student's name and the date, 12 numbered lines to record words, and Jane's name at the bottom. A note of instruction and thanks to the parents is at the top.

Flashlight Game

Children love flashlights! Therefore this old standby of articulation therapy causes much spontaneous speech for activating carryover. Hide speech cards around the therapy room, turn off the lights, and search for them with a flashlight. The activity works best if the room can get fairly dark when the lights are off, so make sure to close blinds or drapes, and arrange furniture for safety. Practice the words before hiding the cards, while searching for them, and after they are found. An activity like this nicely balances drill and spontaneous functional speech. The activity also can be done in a more advanced way without speech cards. Use flashlights to search for regular objects in the room that have their sounds. For little children, hide toys that have their sounds, and practice the words while searching for them. For example, when practicing the word *car*, say, "Where is that car? We need to find that car. Car…! Car…! Where are you, car?"

Fortuneteller Activity

Linda Houge Gustafson submitted a fortuneteller game that she uses for carryover. A *fortuneteller* is a homemade origami game used by children the world over. It also has been called a *cootie catcher*, a *scrunchie*, or a *chatterbox*. A piece of paper is folded in such a way that the item fits on the fingers, and its various flaps can be lifted to reveal messages. One child asks a question, and the other manipulates the fortuneteller. The questioner selects colors and numbers written on the flaps, and these guide the controller in his manipulation of the gadget until it comes to a final answer. [Readers are referred to a friend or the Internet for instructions on constructing a fortuneteller. On the web, search under *paper fortuneteller*.]

The fortuneteller is used to stimulate spontaneous conversation through a simple question-answer format. The questioner poses a question like, "Will I pass my math test today?" The process of finding the answer, and the final answer itself, is read aloud and discussed. The answers (fortunes) make the game fun. Some answers are very specific, others make no sense, and still others are open to interpretation. Linda kindly submitted the following fortunes organized by target phonemes:

R

Keep an open mind but don't let your brains fall out.
Persistence will be rewarded.
You will get what your heart desires.
Rain is in your future. Get an umbrella.
Your kind words will warm someone up today.
You will do the Macarena repeatedly at recess.
Remember the sun always shines after it rains.
You will pour Spot Remover on your dog and make him disappear.
Say, "Rubber baby buggy bumpers" 3 times fast.

S and Z

Someday you will be president.
You can't judge a zebra by its stripes.
See a dentist so fortune will smile on you.
Stop hurrying.
Embrace joy.
Reward yourself.
You will stand up for what's right.
When winds of misfortune blow, go inside.
You will soon play outside.
See a doctor soon.
Pat yourself on the back for doing your best.

Ch and J

You will cheer someone up today.
You will see a chicken cross the road.
You will have intelligent children.
Look up as good fortune will befall you.
You will tell a good joke today.
You will change something today.
You will do something courageous.
Say three times fast, "I want some cheese please Louise."
You will give your teacher a compliment.

Sh

The shorter your fuse, the shorter your life will be.
Friendship is coming.

Shut my flap please, I'm shy!
You used to be indecisive, now you're not sure.
When the sun shines, you will wear sunscreen.
One wish will come true.
Your successes will astonish!
Resist temptation.
You will find a bushel of money.

L

You will use your talents today.
You will give all you can tomorrow.
Brrr…. Put my flap back, I'm cold!
Good luck will smile on you later today.
Someday you will fly to the moon.
You will win a race.
A relative will telephone you.
A hamster will fall in your lap.

K and G

Never cut what you can untie.
You will overcome difficult things.
You will have good luck.
You will receive a compliment today.
Good luck will smile on you later today.
You need to count your blessings.
You will have a good week. (Enjoy it while it lasts).
A bully will appear in your future. You will ignore him.
You will win a game.

F and V

If everyone were a worm, you would be a glowworm.
You will give yourself a bear hug.
You will call a friend.
A relative will send you a gift.
You will try a new food soon.
You will receive a gift soon.
Florescent hair is in your future.
You will be famous.

Th

The best things in life are not things.
You will see that everything has beauty in it.
Your teeth will shine tomorrow.
You will tell your mother or father you love them.

You will thank someone today.
You will earn something today.
Remember, if you mess up, duct tape can fix almost anything.
Do not upset the panther today.
You will get some new clothes soon.

Gathering Signatures

Some therapists have their students gather signatures for carryover. The child is given a special card with a place for 5-10 signatures. The client's job is to go to that many adults during the course of the week and ask for their signature. They explain to the adults that they are collecting signatures for good speech. The adult signs if he or she observes the child using good speech during the day. The cards are returned for reward.

Gifts and Favors

Make gifts and party favors that involve the client's speech targets. Use the activity as a time to work on spontaneous speech. For example, make balloon animals while practicing L, make a Valentine's Day card while practicing V, or make a tongue-depressor picture frame while practicing H in the phrase *Happy Mother's Day!* Design these activities to be completed within one session, or to be worked on a little bit at a time over the course of several weeks. For more simple homemade gift ideas, search the web under *crafts, craft projects, homemade gifts,* and *children's homemade gifts*.

Go Fish

Probably the oldest trick in the book to stimulate spontaneous productions is the game called *Go Fish*. Kids love this old standby. There are professionally made fishing games now, but speech-language pathologists still can make them. I personally like the homemade game because there is so much additional activity and spontaneous talk involved in making the fish and the rods, and because homemade cards are personal to the children. Have the kids draw pictures of their target words on index cards, and put a metal paper clip on each. These cards with their paper clips are the fish. Scatter the fish on the floor. Make a fishing rod from a stick on which is fastened a string. Sticks can be brought in from outside, or use a doll rod, a firm straw, or a chopstick. Fasten a small magnet on the end of the string. The magnet will attract the paper clips and function as a hook. Fish for the cards by dangling the magnet near the paper clips. Name the fish that are caught. Place the caught fish in a box or bowl. Encourage spontaneous conversation throughout.

Grading Charts

Alicia Roberts has established *Grading Charts* in therapy to help her clients develop self-discrimination and to show them how to become their own therapists. The clients rate their own productions as *Great, Okay,* or *Do Over*. Next to each rating they write down what constitutes this category. Descriptions are done in the client's own words. Pictures are used with young clients. For example:

- GREAT: Here they spell out exactly what makes for an excellent production, like, "The sound came out the middle."
- OKAY: Here they spell out what makes a production just okay, like, "It sounds weird."
- DO OVER: Here they spell out what makes it necessary for the client to try again, like, "The sound came out the sides."

Grocery Shopping

Grocery shopping makes for an excellent carryover activity for parents because it is such a common and recurring activity. Have the parent work together with the child to generate the shopping list, identify all the words that have their target sound, and practice the words at home or on the way to the store. Then allow the actual shopping experience be the time during which spontaneous productions of the words ensue. Consider having the parents encourage other methods for correction during the shopping experience. For example, tell them to have the client tally his correct or incorrect utterances with a clicker counter in the store. Allow the child a grocery store treat like candy or popsicles for achieving a certain number of correct spontaneous productions during the shopping experience. This way the child will go out of his way to say targets frequently.

Hallway Walks

Stacey Misko promotes carryover by stimulating the client to practice during the time he walks to and from therapy. She uses poster-tack to hang articulation cards on the wall in the hall that leads to her therapy room. The client views the cards on the way to and from therapy. The hanging pictures are considered artwork hanging in a gallery. During the walk, the client has to say the sound, word, phrase, or sentence that goes with the picture. He also has to define the word by giving three attributes of the picture. Another idea Stacey uses for hall practice is to put dots or footprints on the wall or floor so that clients have to produce their targets each time they pass or step on one as they walk down the hall.

Hidden Pictures

Children usually love to search through drawings for hidden images. I use the ones that appear in *Highlights* magazines for children. Those pictures alone are worth the subscription price. Sometimes I make these drawings up myself, or the kids make them and challenge their friends to find the hidden picture. Much conversation is generated while searching for and designing hidden images. Also, everyone is familiar with the *Where's Waldo* book series and the challenge of finding Waldo in his amazing scenes. Other books similar to this are being published today. I always keep hidden picture drawings and books in my therapy room to contrast with other work that may be boring.

High-Tech Alarms

Amy Lang finds that usually it is the parent who forgets to do the child's carryover activities at home, and she is using the new technologies to help them remember. For example, she may have a parent set their cell phone alarm to ring while driving the kids to school as a reminder to expect good speech from her child. A text reminder also may be sent. She also has her e-mail program send automatic reminders home. Some therapists use these alarms with their students too.

Homemade Books

Many therapists submitted ideas about making books for carryover. Use pages the children draw themselves, copy pages from other published workbooks, print pictures found on the Internet, or cut photographs and other images from magazines to paste on paper. Use regular blank photocopy paper, stack the pages, and then staple them at least three times along one side to bind them together like a book. Most children absolutely love to make books, even when their drawings are primitive and their handwriting looks like chicken scratches. Children can share these books with parents, grandparents, and others who visit the home. This is an excellent carryover idea that dovetails with literacy. Create one book for every individual purpose or skill. As examples:

- Make an individual book of a target phoneme in all positions of words.
- Make an individual book of a target phoneme represented in only one target position. Make other books for other positions.
- Make a book that revolves around one single target word or phrase.
- Make a book that revolves around a series of target words or phrases.

For example, Amy Schuchman helps her clients who are working on Th to create a book called *Theo the Python Slithers on the Path.* Theo travels along the path and has various encounters along the way. For example, he finds *three teeth* and a *moth taking a bath.* Amy writes out the words as the client draws the pictures.

Homemade Flipbooks

Kim Watson-Setliff makes homemade flipbooks during the last five minutes of therapy as a way to wrap up the session and have something to take away for carryover. She uses large (5x7 inch) blank index cards stapled together on the left-hand side to make the book. She writes the child's name and sound on the front, for example, *Elena's L Book.* She uses scissors to cut the first page three inches from the right-hand side, the second page 2.5 inches from the right, the third page 2 inches from the right, and so forth. This makes the first page the shortest and the last page the longest for easy flipping. On each page is drawn a picture or a word, or some other content related to the therapy done in session that day. A story can be portrayed from page to page. She also may write a reading log at the end so the flipbook can be used in conjunction with classroom reading requirements. Books are made all throughout the course of the year, so by the end of the year the client has a substantial library of little homemade flipbooks that can be read at home or during non-structured times in the classroom. She makes the books for the little children but has older students construct their own. I love this idea!

Host a Party

Plan a birthday, holiday, or special occasion party. Use the planning time to find and rehearse words with speech targets. Use the kids' target sounds in the preparation of accoutrements, practice party talk and party games, and make party invitations and little gifts that incorporate target sounds. Have the party and discuss the outcome. Planning and hosting a party may be one of the most normal carryover activities we can do with children. Host pretend parties for dolls and stuffed animals in situations where other children are not available.

Hot and Cold Game

Shirley Schindeldecker submitted an excellent game for carryover that she says her children love. This is a game to play in the therapy room and to send home. Make a 5x5 box grid, and write a target word in each box. Give one player 6 colored chips. The other players secretly select one word from the grid that they write down on a separate paper and hide from sight. The person with the chips now looks at the grid of words and asks questions to guess which one they selected. He asks, "Are you thinking of___?" The children in the group respond, "No, we are not thinking of___. You are hot (or cold)." The word *hot* is used if the word asked about is adjacent to the target square. The word *cold* is use if the word asked about is not touching the target square. The questioning continues until the selected word is discovered. The child with the chips has to give up one chip for each incorrect guess. The person with the most chips at the end wins!

Huge Pictures

I use large rolls of butcher-type paper to make huge wall pictures that the children and I draw together. I have always found this to be a fabulous way to generate spontaneous speech. Place the paper on the floor, or on a huge table cleared of all other material. Let the children draw spontaneously and let the topic of the picture go where it will. Incorporate therapy words into the theme. Use colorful markers or watercolor paints. Write the target words on the picture and give it a title. Hang the artwork on the wall in the hall for all to marvel over and talk about.

Ice Cream Sundaes

Here's a great idea for kids who need to get fired up about carryover. Make ice cream sundaes! Jackie Zuelke-Karch did this with a group of boys. The idea was for the boys to serve ice cream sundaes to others by acting as servers and asking their customers what type of ice cream they want, which ingredients they desire, and so forth. First they practiced with pictures to create scripts. Then they used a plastic ice cream set to role-play with each other. Then she arranged ahead of time for certain adults to come to the room to order real sundaes. Their homework was to do the same activity at home with their families.

Index Cards

A deck of blank index cards probably is one of the most useful items in the carryover process, especially for young children who love to pretend play. Have kids develop their own decks of cards by drawing pictures with colorful markers. Write the target word below the picture. Therapists everywhere use these cards to create play activities in order to stimulate spontaneous speech. For example:

- ROADS: Use the cards to build roads on which tiny cars and trucks drive, and to fashion sidewalks on which small dolls and other figures walk.

- LOADS: Use the cards as loads while playing with dump trucks. Name the cards while loading and dumping. Move piles from one end of the room to the other. Talk about the loads and their transportation.
- MAIL: Use the cards as mail to place in toy mailboxes. Use a shoebox if you don't have a mailbox.
- PLACEMATS: Use the cards as placemats for doll tea parties. Set the table and have the party.
- ART: Use the cards as art to fasten to a bulletin board. Have an art show. Role-play the curators and patrons.
- CLOTHES: Pretend the cards are clothes and role-play laundry day. Use one box as a washer and another as a dryer. Pin the cards to a clothesline to dry. Place the clothes neatly in a dresser drawer. Punch holes in the cards in order to hang the clothes onto real hangers.
- MONEY: Role-play a shopping experience. Use the cards as cash for making purchases in a store. Stock the store with play food and other toys.

Internet Topics

As everyone knows today, the Internet is an amazing tool to find information on just about any topic under the sun. If you have a computer in your therapy room and are on-line, the clients can search for just about any topic for discussion. For example, if the client is working on R, use the Internet to look up how to build a robot. Also consider having the client look this up at home as a homework activity, and then come to therapy the next time with a printout of the things he has found. In groups, have each child bring information they have found at home, and then have them read or tell about it to the group. Consider having each member of the group look up the same topic and then talk among themselves to find how the information they obtained was the same or different. [Warning: Do not assign homework activities in which children search topics related to the mouth such as *lips, jaw,* or *tongue*. These key words draw many inappropriate sites. Stick to safer child friendly topics.]

Jigsaw Puzzles

Many therapists use jigsaw puzzles to induce spontaneous speech. If you have worked on jigsaw puzzles at home with your family, you know that this can be a silent activity as people concentrate on the process of constructing the puzzle. But usually there is some discussion that runs along certain lines. Often questions are asked about the size and shape of the pieces — "Have you seen a piece that is flat on one side and has a huge bump on the other?" Begin by encouraging the children to talk about the process of puzzle building, and then let the puzzle be a background for all manner of talk. Keep puzzles of various difficulty levels in your room to challenge children of all ages and cognitive levels, from simple 3-piece form puzzles to 100-piece jigsaw puzzles. If your therapy room allows it, you may even have a permanent working area for a 1000-piece puzzle.

Joke of the Day

Renee Berg has her clients tell the family one joke per day. This is a great carryover activity that clients will look forward to everyday. Clients who do not remember jokes well may need to jot them down in a little journal or on index cards. Younger siblings will beg for more when these jokes are told at home. A speech therapy room for elementary age students is incomplete without a joke book. Search the web for children's jokes.

Journals

Some therapists give journals to their clients to write in at home as a carryover activity. The clients record many things in the journal during the week between sessions. They might write down troublesome words they encounter during the week, activities during which they successfully produced target sounds, a list of people with whom they tried their new sounds, the scores for word games played with family members, a tally of errors made during a reading activity, and so forth. Purchase nice journals at dollar stores and garage sales, or purchase tiny 50¢ spiral notebooks.

Key Word Questionnaire

Stacey R. Honowitz has a procedure for obtaining key words from the family. She sends home a questionnaire for the parents to clearly write the full names of the people in the child's life whose names should be used in speech activities. The questionnaire has a place to record the correct spelling of the student's name, as well as the names of the parents, siblings, special friends, pets, relatives, neighbors, friends, activity leaders, and other important folk. She uses these supplied names in some of her earliest activities, and these names remain with them throughout the program. Stacey reports that her students seem honored to use these names in their work with her. I really like this activity because it shows the parents right away that you care about their family, and it helps them realize that you are working on things that matter.

Lending Library

Beth Marafiote carefully organizes her own collection of Scholastic's *Step Into Reading* books to send home as carryover activities for preschool children. She sends the children home with a book that has some words with their sound of the week, and the children are to pretend to read the book to their parents every day. Some books are easy while others are a little harder. Some have more of a specific target sound while others contain the target only a few times. Knowing the basic information about each book allows her to pick one for the child's level of production. Beth's clients and their parents report that they love this form of homework. The books allow both the parents and the child to anticipate the sound, and books also develop parent-child bonding, language development, and literacy enhancement.

The children keep only one book at a time in this lending library activity, and they only get a new book when they return the one they borrowed. That way the books are not lost. Beth finds that she does lose two or three books per year, but reports that parents often offer to replace them. She has found that she has to stop giving books to certain families because the books consistently come back destroyed. Beth keeps an index card clipped inside each book. The index card has the book name, author, and number on it. Then she writes the child's name and borrowing date on the card. The card is put in an envelope, and these envelopes are organized by the day of the week. The index cards allow her to tell parents what book they have out when they forget to bring it back. She knows how long they have had the book since the index card is dated. Putting the author on the index card also allows her to order another one easily when necessary.

Marafiote has been operating her lending library for 15 years while working with over 700 children, and she has collected about 180 books. Each book is numbered and the number is recorded on a poster-size master sheet hanging next to the bookshelf. The master sheet lists all of the target sounds vertically, and each sound is represented twice—for initial and final position. Each time she purchases a new book, she numbers it, and then studies it to determine which sounds are exemplified best. Then she writes the book number on the chart next to the target sound for which it can be used. When she needs to pick a book for a child, she first scans down the chart for the target sound, and then scans across for book numbers. This allows her to select appropriate carryover books quickly. I love this idea! Beth uses a letter to introduce the lending library to her families. It says:

> I would like to start a *Lending Library* with your child. I will give your child a book that is to be returned the following week. A new book will then be traded for the returned book. The book will have some words that contain the sound your child is working on that week. The purpose of these books is to help your child bridge the gap between correctly producing sounds at the word or sentence level to producing them accurately in conversation. Many of the books are easy enough for your child to memorize most of the text.
>
> After you read the book to your child a few times, he is to 'read' it back to you. It is 'Speech Time' and your child has to pronounce the sounds accurately. Saying the exact text is not important. Have your child correct his sound errors. Praise his accurate productions. If your child has trouble retelling the story to you, ask questions that elicit sentence responses. For example, say, 'Tell me what is happening in this picture.' Try to have your child 'read' the book once daily. Remember, you want <u>your child to tell the story</u> to help carry-over of newly learned sounds to conversation.

Library Visits

Most children have library teaching activities incorporated into their school programs, and this is an excellent place where articulation carryover can work into the curriculum. Initiate a library activity in which the client's target phoneme becomes the key element of a search. For example, pick a key word like *zebra* if the client is working on Z. Use this word as the foundation of any number of activities, for example:

- Use the library's search engine to find all the books in the library about zebras.
- Use the library's search engine to find a few books about zebras and read them together.
- Use the library's search engine to make a master list of all the books with the word *zebra* in the title.
- Use the library's search engine to make a master list of all books that contain information about zebras.
- Search through encyclopedias for information about zebras.
- Browse through the shelves of children's picture books and guess which ones have zebras in them by analyzing the books by title and cover artwork. Search through the

books to see if you were right.
- Have the client talk to the librarian about how to find a book about zebras.
- Have the client report to his group, his class, or his parents how he accomplished any of the activities above.

Loaded Sentences

Janet Robinson has her students see how many target words they can load into one single sentence. This makes long and nonsensical sentences that children adore. Here's an example for R: *Rufus Radcliff rooted rapidly inside a red car after really rotten roosters ran recklessly after radical rats*. Some therapists make the activity more challenged by disallowing *and* as a conjunction.

Loaded Speech Monologues

This is a game to build control in rapid conversational speech. Each child is given 30 seconds to speak on a selected topic. The children are challenged to put as many target words into their monologues as possible. The other children tally the number of target words that are used. The child with the highest number wins. The time limit forces the kids to speak fast and furiously, and most kids end up saying crazy things just to cram words into their speech. I usually let the kids use the conjunction *and.* For example, when working on S and S-clusters, a client might say, "I like to go skating because squirrels skate fast, and my sister skates fast, and so sixteen is her age, and soon she will be seventeen, and so Sam likes snakes, and sponges are sopping wet, and stale bread is sticky!"

Mad Libs

Therapists who submitted ideas for this book mentioned the game of *Mad Libs* so often that it deserves its own section. The name of the game is an adaptation of the term *ad lib*, which in modern theater means *spontaneous improvision* (from the Latin *ab libitum* meaning *at one's pleasure*). In the game, one player prompts another for a list of words to substitute for blanks in a story. The one who supplies the words does not know the story ahead of time; therefore the story becomes hilarious when read aloud. Leonard Stern and Roger Price published their first Mad Libs book in 1958, and others published today are available at bookstores and through children's book clubs. Therapists use them by substituting therapy word targets for the blanks. Playing this game can cause much laughter and spontaneous speech in the session.

Magnets, Magnetic Toys, and Magnetic Play Sets

Children are fascinated with magnets and playing with them can create a wonderful setting for spontaneous speech. I have always kept a small box of magnets and metal objects in a drawer to pull out at that special moment when therapy needs a little light-hearted boost. Keep paper clips, hairpins, nuts and bolts, screws and nails, bits of wire and metal pieces found here and there in the box. Keep the small round magnets from used shower curtains. Magnetic wands and other magnetic toys also are available, and magnetic scene toys are favorites among the elementary set. Magnet play can be so fascinating that children remain quiet while discovering their properties, so think about how you are going to add speech work into the activity. I usually let the kids play freely with the magnets for a while before I add in the speech requirements.

Mail Delivery

Several therapists submitted ideas about mail delivery activities. Most said that they arrange with their school to allow certain speech students to deliver mail to the teachers. For example, a student may hand-deliver a flyer about an upcoming meeting to each teacher in the building instead of having the secretary place one in each teacher's mailbox. The therapist and student write a script for delivery ahead of time. The script contains multiple instances of the target sound. Some therapists have their clients also hand a performance evaluation card to each teacher so they can check a box to rate the student's performance. Follow-up discussion ensues in the therapy session.

Manicures

I have used manicures to facilitate spontaneous speech with just the right clients. I usually ask the children if they are interested and then send home a permission slip about it. Stimulus words can be practiced ahead of time, and the activity can be role-played first. The actual nail-painting ceremony is used to stimulate spontaneous productions of target sounds. Color words for working on R fit in nicely here because there are so many different red nail colors — dark red, light red, cherry red, rose red, pale red, red apple, red cranberry, and so forth. Nails also can be painted with shapes to make red and white stripes, half red and half black, red with yellow dots, and so forth. This is a great activity to do one-on-one, with a speech buddy, or at home.

Memory / Match Game for Home

Every therapist plays memory and matching games in therapy and most of us have beautiful card sets with which to do so. Kim Marty Smoot suggested an easy way to send home cards for the family to play these games. She makes two copies each of her articulation cards. She then sends them home for the family to cut into card size and to play the games. Parents can get these laminated, or they can buy clear plastic shelving paper and cover them themselves.

Monitoring Sheets

Many therapists wrote about forms they have developed for self-monitoring. Zina Santos has developed a *Speech Monitoring Sheet* that she gives her middle-school students. The students choose one class in which to monitor their speech. They are to use the sheet to comment on how they did during the class. Responses include: Good, Better, Okay, I forgot, I didn't talk today, and so forth. There is also a box on the form for the child to write down words that were difficult. After the child has used the form in one class, the work is increased to two classes, and so forth. The sheet also contains a box for home activities like riding in the car or eating dinner. The clients are rewarded for completing their sheets.

Morning Announcements and Pledge

Many therapists make arrangements with their schools to have speech students read morning announcements or to recite the Pledge of Allegiance on the public address system. Students practice ahead of time with the therapist. The performances are recorded if possible for study in the next speech class. Students often grade their own performances of this carryover activity.

Mottos

Grace Medina-Chow teaches her clients speech mottos to stimulate carryover. Mottos are slogans or sayings that express a rule by which to live. For example, she teaches her clients that *practice is everywhere*. In every session she also asks, "When do you practice your speech?" The clients respond, "All the time!"

Music Conductor

Karen Larssen has her clients act like orchestra or choral conductors as they lead speech production activities in their small groups. One child stands in front of the group and uses his arms and hands to direct the others. He gestures to the group members to say their target sounds or words individually or together in unison. The conductor sets the rhythm and creates the masterpieces. Great idea. Musical students, and those who like to be in charge, would love this.

Ned's Head, Feeler Boxes, Bags, and Socks

The game that was mentioned more than any other by contributing speech-language pathologists was the popular game called *What's in Ned's Head?* The game includes a big stuffed head that has open orifices (mouth, ears) into which tiny toys and other objects can be hidden. The children reach into an opening and try to guess what the object is before they pull it out. Kids love this.

Before the manufacturing of this popular game, speech-language pathologists used to make *Feeler Boxes* out of shoeboxes. Cut a hole into each of the four sides of a shoebox. Make the holes large enough for a child's hand to fit inside. Cover each hole with a piece of cloth or felt. Hide an object in the box that the child has to feel and guess. Every therapist used to make one of these boxes to work with children. I think I still have one out in my garage that I made in graduate school. Even a paper bag or a sock cinched at the top can be employed when Ned's Head is not available. Save money by improvising.

News Stories

Many therapists use current news stories for reading material, prepared presentations, and spontaneous speech. Printed news articles are chosen and words are highlighted. The published articles are read aloud, then the material is organized into a television or radio broadcast to be presented to the group, the class, or taped for later presentation. The material also can be used as a topic for a talk show, and then again later in a spontaneous discussion of current events. This activity can be done in conjunction with any number of classroom topics depending upon the chosen news topic. Donna McDonough also uses radio and television news stories to develop auditory awareness of target sounds. Clients listen to real news broadcasts at home and jot down the words they hear broadcasters say that have their sounds. Then they give the news themselves later in speech or in their classroom.

Parent Information Sheets

Many therapists develop information sheets to send home to parents for carryover. The sheets contain basic information about what sound(s) the child is currently working on, along with a list of simple ways they can reinforce the child's productions at home. Any of the activities in this book could be included on these lists. Therapists should feel free to photocopy any of these pages to send home for parents.

Photocopying

The easiest way to send therapy material home for speech carryover is to photocopy the professional speech cards you already are using with the clients in therapy. A fast and powerful photocopier can be very expensive and take up a lot of space in a therapy room or office. But there are simple solutions for this. First, if you have a computer and printer in your room, the printer might have a copy function as well. Second, an old fax machine usually can make copies. For years I had an old fax machine that I used as my office phone and as a copier. I think I bought it for $10 at a thrift store. An old fax machine copies much more slowly than a modern photocopier, but the slow copying routine can make time for further nice discussions. Usually 4–6 speech cards can fit onto one single paper for copying. Fasten cards with a dab of rubber cement so that the cards can be removed from the paper and the glue can be rubbed off afterwards. (You don't want to ruin your nice speech cards in the process.) The copy can be left intact as a full 8.5x11-inch sheet, or the individual pictures can be cut to be card size. I always have left my copies in the page format so they can be punched with three holes and placed in the client's three-ring speech binder for carrying home.

Photographs

Some therapists use photographs to promote carryover. Leah Christianson buys inexpensive photo frames and places a photograph of the client in the frame. The photo shows the client holding a sign that reads, "I will say my ___ sound the new way." The children place the frames somewhere they will see them often. Jill Richards uses her digital camera to take photos of her clients holding toys or objects that start with their target sounds. These are made into picture books to take home.

Pick-a-Night

Mary Meehan has a good idea for organizing the way good speech is encouraged during conversations at home. She has the family pick one night a week during which the child is to use his corrected sounds during a conversation. No correction needs to be made during the conversation, but the parent and child discuss it privately later in the evening. They talk about how they think the conversation went. If things go well, then two nights are selected, then three, and so on.

Picture Drawing Guessing Game

This game requires one child to draw while another gives instructions. The child giving the instructions knows what is to be drawn, but the child with the writing utensil doesn't. The child giving instructions must use good speech while giving the other child simple instructions, and he must not use any specific instructions. For example, he cannot say, "Draw a car." Instead he must say, "Draw a horizontal line in the middle of the page… Now draw a circle under the line on one end, touching the line… Now draw another one on the other side of the line…" The drawer has to guess what he's drawing. The children can be timed to see who gets their idea across fastest.

Placemats

Several speech-language pathologists who responded to our call for ideas suggested the making of placemats for home carryover stimulation. Purchase inexpensive placemats, or make your own out of construction paper. The children draw or fasten pictures to them, and target sounds and words are written on the mats. The mats are laminated and the children take them home to use as a daily reminder during meals and snacks. This is a simple idea that will impact children daily. I love it because it is so old-fashioned and home friendly.

Playdough Creations

Cheryl Lunny reminds us that children love Playdough, and that creating with Playdough is an excellent way to stimulate spontaneous speech. There is something about the color, texture, and smell of Playdough that is simply irresistible to children and adults alike. I have always kept cookie cutters and modeling tools for the children to use as they create with Playdough. Cheryl suggests to have the kids use their target sounds as they talk about all the creations. For example, if Ch were the target sound, then the word *dinosaur* would be called a "Chinosaur" and so forth.

Play Money

Many therapists use play money called *SpeechBucks* that students can earn for participation in homework and carryover activities. The children are paid when they turn in carryover assignments. SpeechBucks are used to purchase items in the treasure box or to earn some other privilege. This is straight behavior modification at it most simple and practical. The earned SpeechBucks can be kept in the therapist's room in special individual envelopes to make sure they are not lost. Some therapists give SpeechBucks to classroom teachers and parents to dole out at appropriate times. Another idea is to operate a speech checking or savings account instead of using actual play money. Use bank checking or savings account registers, or set up mock accounts on the computer. Use the accounts to accumulate and spend money for speech words.

Play Models

I use play sets to stimulate spontaneous speech. For example, I have a McDonald's restaurant play set complete with Ronald, a drive through window, and a family. I have added a car and some tiny play food to complete the experience. Children adore playing with this set and it encourages much spontaneous play throughout. I even use it with older children who like to fiddle with the pieces as they talk about their own McDonald's experiences.

Plays

Many therapists who responded to our carryover activity survey wrote about the use of plays for stimulating carryover. Acting out a play is a common sense idea for carryover that has been with us for a very long time, and even some of our earliest books recommended using plays to take new speech skills to their ultimate performance mode. Plays can be performed in the speech class, or they can be performed in front of a whole class or an entire school. The need to project the voice well, to control rate, and to pronounce with clarity make acting a very important way to develop expressive speech and carryover. The public nature of the play makes it a wonderful bridge from words to conversation.

Positive Notes for Parents

An excellent way to promote carryover at home is to take a few minutes to write a positive note to the parents about how well their child is doing. Write the note in front of the child as he watches and waits. Be bold and up front about this. Consider reading the note out loud as you write it, or ask the client to read it out loud to you once you have finished it. For example, write, "Johnny did great today. He can say S correctly now. Ask him to show you how he is doing it. Have him say 'supper' for you. He can do it perfectly!"

Preschool Homework

Philip Shively reminds us that preschool children love to be given homework especially if they see older brothers and sisters occupied with such in the evenings. Philip uses a computer program in which he can make pages of pictures and words. These pages, and other workbook pages pulled from here and there, become the child's homework for practice with parents. The children can color the pictures, circle the words, and so forth.

Propaganda (Influencing the Physical Environment)

Some writers have suggested that the therapy room itself should suggest good speech as a motivating factor in carryover. Today we might call this *influencing the physical environment*, but it has been called *propaganda* in prior decades: "Propaganda for good speech will be an aid to motivation and carryover" (Powers, 1971, p. 900). Powers suggested that we decorate our speech rooms with posters and a display of newspaper or magazine articles about people who have good speech, people who have given good speeches, or people who have overcome speech or hearing deficits. Classroom teachers do this all the time by decorating their bulletin boards with people who represent certain concepts; therefore this is an untested yet very common teaching method. Here are a few examples of important people with speech and hearing impairment that were found through a simple browsing of the Internet:

- LUDWIG VAN BEETHOVEN: Classical music composer with hearing impairment.
- CURTIS PRIDE: Professional baseball player with hearing impairment.
- KENNY WALKER: Professional football player with hearing impairment.
- JULIETTE LOW: Founder of Girl Scouts of America with hearing impairment.
- HEATHER WHITESTONE MCCALLUM: The only Miss America with hearing impairment.
- RUSH LIMBAUGH: Number one daytime talk radio host with hearing impairment who wears a cochlear implant.
- DOUGLAS TILDEN: Bronze sculptor with hearing impairment.

- MICHELLE BANKS: Modern day performer with hearing impairment.
- MARLEE MATLIN: Modern day actress who with hearing impairment.
- RONALD REAGAN: 40th U.S. President with hearing impairment who wore hearing aids.
- LOU FERRIGNO: Bodybuilder and actor with hearing impairment.
- JOHN GLENN: First American astronaut to orbit the Earth who has a history of stuttering.
- CARLY SIMON: Singer-song writer with a history of stuttering.
- JAMES EARL JONES: Modern day actor who has a history of stuttering.
- BRUCE WILLIS: Modern day actor with a history of stuttering.
- STEPHEN HAWKING: Theoretical physicist who has Lou Gehrig's disease and uses augmentative communication.
- CHRISTY BROWN: Writer with cerebral palsy and severe dysarthria (*My Left Foot*, 1954).

Question Games

Designing activities in which clients must ask questions has always been a favorite way of stimulating spontaneous speech. For example, Paula Groothuis uses laminated cards or pictures. She places a sticker on the back of one card, then the cards are placed face-up on the table so the location of the sticker is a mystery. Any number of pictures can be used, but a limit of ten is appropriate for most elementary age children. The children have to guess which card has the sticker by asking, "Is the sticker on the back of the ___?" This question becomes more loaded with target phonemes as therapy advances. For example, in advanced stages of R therapy, a sticker of a girl might be used and the question might be, "Is the <u>picture</u> of the <u>girl</u> behind the <u>car</u>?"

Random Number Generators

A fun way to encourage spontaneous production of the numbers is to use a random number generator. A random number generator is a computer program that draws a number randomly. Search on the Internet under *random number generators*. There are a variety of them that are easy to use. Most require you simply to select the number of random numbers you want generated and to select the range. For example, you may want the program to generate ten numbers between the numbers of 50 and 300. The computer automatically will give you ten randomly selected numbers from this range. Learn how to use one of these sites yourself first, and then make an activity where you show the client how to do it. Talk through the whole process. Use the random number generator by itself for fun and practice, or use it for some purpose, like deciding which page to read in a textbook.

Recordings — Audio or Video

Many therapists who responded to our call for carryover activities submitted ideas about making audio or video recordings of clients in various performances. The material is selected and rehearsed, and then performed for the camera or audio recording equipment. The recordings can be heard or viewed in therapy, and they can be sent home for homework or family entertainment. Video recordings can be shown in the classroom, or they can be used in an assembly for the whole school. Videos also can be posted on the Internet with appropriate parent permission. Audio recordings can be transferred to MP3 capable phones for home listening. Do this all with home recorders, or go on a field trip to a local recording studio willing to donate an hour of their time. Be careful not to loose the focus on the speech tasks while otherwise engaged in these exciting activities. Examples follow:

- TEACHING VIDEOS: Judith Lunger-Bergh makes teaching videos in which clients teach a skill such as *How to Decorate a Cookie*, or *How to Peel and Eat an Orange without Making a Huge Mess*, or *How to Make Thumb Print Characters*.
- SPEECH TRAINING TAPES: Record clients teaching about speech therapy. Use topics such as *How to Make the R Sound*, *How to Use Bingo in Speech Class*, or *How to Play 'I Spy' in the Car to Practice Your Speech with Your Family.*
- CLASSIC PLAYS: Record the children acting out a scene from a classic play.
- NEW MINI-DRAMAS: Record the children in a short drama of their own creation. Use target words as the basis of a mini-drama created by the children with therapist guidance.
- READING: Record the clients as they read. For example, record them as they read paragraphs from their own novels or textbooks. Also record them as they read children's picture books to be shown in classrooms of younger children. Or record them as they read their own prose or poetry to be submitted to a writing contest.
- INTERVIEWS: Record clients interviewing one another, or have the clients interview a special child in the school, such as the captain of the volleyball team or the winner of an essay contest. Interview an adult in the school such as a teacher, principal, school nurse, or a secretary. Also consider having the children interview a local celebrity like the mayor, a local television news reporter, the owner of a popular restaurant, and so forth.
- ADVERTISEMENTS: Produce a television or radio advertisement. Make one up or reproduce one the kids have already seen.
- NEWS REPORTING: Record a mock news program. Use national, local, family, or school news.
- STAND-UP COMEDY: Record the clients telling jokes or doing prepared stand-up comedy routines.
- MUSIC: Record the children singing. Or record the clients introducing themselves or others who will play a musical selection on an instrument.
- CHARACTER VOICES: Children love simply to hear their own voices on an audio recording, and making character voices can enhance this activity. Have the kids try to make the voice of Elmer Fudd, Bugs Bunny, or Donald Duck. Try Elmo, Big Bird, or Oscar the Grouch.
- ACCENTS: Record your clients as they attempt accents while maintaining correct speech. Discuss the differences between phonemes as they are spoken in various languages. For example, discuss the differences between R as it is spoken in English, French, Spanish, and Japanese. Also discuss the variations on R spoken in English in the countries of Britain, Ireland, Scotland, Australia, New Zealand, and in various regions in the United States.

Rehearse and Do

Vivian Binnington reminds us that carryover can be stimulated by having clients practice their sounds or words while doing other activities. For example, have the client practice targets while hopping, walking, running, or while following a direction like, "Bring me the blue book on the top shelf." Make the work more difficult by having the client continue to rehearse while carrying out a series of steps, like tying a pair of shoes, or washing and drying the hands. Vivian reports that she used to hold back this activity until clients were consistently accurate at the word level, but over time she began to include it in therapy right from the beginning. She asks, "Why wait?"

Reinforcement Phrases

Crystal Luk encourages teachers and caregivers to use specially designed reinforcement phrases to stimulate articulation carryover in the classroom and at home. Each phrase reiterates the child's target phonemes. The teacher or parent says the words and uses the appropriate hand signals that most of us know. Each can be used by itself or in sequence.

- Th — *Thumbs up!* (Give the thumbs up signal).
- B — *Fist bump!* (Bump each other's fists together).
- F — *High five!* (Give the high five signal)
- G — *Good job!* (Touch each other's thumbs).
- O — *Okay!* (Give the classic signal).
- H — *Hip-hop-hooray!* (Raise both hands for a High Ten).
- L — *Low, low, low!* (Child's right hand reaches low to clap the adult's left hand).
- N — *Knuckle bump!* (Bump fisted knuckles together).
- S — *On the side!* (Slap hands together horizontally).
- S-blends — *Smart choice!* (Touch thumb to thumb).
- F, S, D, L, SL — *Give me five, on the side, down low, too slow* (Use all appropriate gestures).

Role-Playing

Speech-language pathologists always have used roll playing as a way to work on spontaneous speech. In a role-playing situation, the setting and situation are determined, but the conversation unfolds spontaneously. For example, the setting might be a dentist office and the situation might be that the child is making an appointment. Key words can be listed to guide the conversation into target sounds. A wide variety of settings can be used in role-playing, for example, restaurants, cafeterias, libraries, movie theaters, birthday parties, soccer practice, piano lessons, and so forth.

Role Reversal

Lynn-Rachel Ary reminds us that role reversal is an excellent way to stimulate carryover. Have the client take the role of speech teacher while you take the role of student. The client pretends to teach the adult how to make a sound, or teaches you a game or activity to be played. This is a nice way to solidify a client's knowledge about what he is doing in therapy.

Routine Family Phrases

Don't forget that many families employ a set of phrases they use to name routine events in the family, and these can be used for carryover training. For example, in my home, when my children were in elementary school, every Friday night was a time for *Friday Night Shows*. That meant that the kids had to clean their rooms after school on Fridays, and they were rewarded with pizza, Pepsi, and four half-hour sit-coms that ran from 8:00 to 10:00. (Not the healthiest choice, I realize, but it kept their rooms clean and made the kids happy.) The phrase *Friday Night Shows* came up all during the week, and it would have been a perfect phrase for carryover of several consonant phonemes — F, R, D, N, T, Sh, and S. Let your students tell you what types of activities like this are used in their homes, or send home a questionnaire about this for the parents to complete. Establish a way for parents to encourage and monitor these productions at home.

Scavenger Hunts

Many therapists use scavenger hunts to promote carryover in school programs. Scavenger hunts are designed so that the speech students have to go from person-to-person in the school in order to accomplish some task. For example:

- OBJECT HUNTS: Give the students a list of things they must find in the school that can be carried in a backpack back to speech class. The list will contain words that have target sounds. For example, in working on S, the list might include *scissors, stapler, eraser, stars, sticky tape,* and *stamps*. Students will have to talk to the teachers and staff from whom they are borrowing the items. Develop a way for the students to record which item came from which adult so they can be returned afterwards.
- CLUE HUNTS: Give written clues to various adults in the school. Give the client the first clue that will lead him to the first adult who also has a clue. That clue leads to the next adult, and so forth. The last person's clue leads the client to the reward or activity.
- RIDDLE HUNTS: This hunt is like the others, but this time each adult has a riddle. The answer to the riddle leads the client to the next adult who has the next riddle, and so forth.
- QUESTION AND ANSWER HUNTS: Write out a series of questions that only certain people in the school will know. The students have to figure out within their group to whom to go to get the answers. For example, the card might read, "Find out the name of the principal's oldest daughter."

School Curriculum Material

We hardly need to say this today: Carryover is more assured when practice material is drawn from the student's curriculum material. Using school curriculum material always has been considered one of the best ways to make speech work functional for the stimulation of carryover: "I believe that an inexhaustible supply of material can be derived from the school curriculum … automaticity of production under conditions wherein attention must be focused on content is the ultimate goal" (Gerber, 1973, p. 60). Have children bring their textbooks to speech on occasion, and talk to the teacher about key words and spelling words. Keep in mind, however, that classroom vocabulary is not controlled by phonetic environment and therefore should not be viewed as a place to begin working on a phoneme. Curriculum material is some of the final material of articulation therapy and therefore it is appropriate for the carryover process.

Scrambled Sentences Game

Gerber (1973) recommended a nice activity using scrambled sentences to be used with children who can read. Write individual sentences with scrambled word order on cards. Give each client a card, and allow 10-20 seconds for them to unscramble the words to make a sentence. Then let the children read the unscrambled sentences to the others. Assign points for unscrambling the sentences and for reading them aloud without error. Let the clients judge one another. Make it even more fun by having the clients make up the scrambled sentences themselves to challenge one another. Increase the speed of the activity by rewarding the first to unscramble his sentence. Increase the frenetic pace by having the children go through the unscrambling process aloud.

Scrambled Sentences Group Game

This game is a take-off on the idea by Gerber above to use in a group of older children. Make one card with one sentence on it per student. Jumble the words, but this time jumble them around from card-to-card so that some words from each sentence are written on each card. That way each student holds a card with words that belong to himself and to every other student. The children have to speak to one another and sort out which words really belong on which cards to make intelligent sentences. Divide the children into two teams to increase the competitiveness. The sentences are read aloud once the words are sorted. By the way, there might be more than one way to sort the words, thus making the activity even more interesting.

Sensory Tables

Many therapists use sensory tables or sensory boxes to stimulate spontaneous speech. Fill the box or sensory table with smooth dried beans such as kidneys, limas, lentils, or pintos. Hide toys in the beans for the children to search for with their hands. Most children love this. Use toys with target phonemes in the names, and talk about them as the children are searching. Reverse roles and let the children hide toys for you to discover too. Plastic toys also can be hidden in tubs of bubbly water. Make sure the bubbles are thick enough to conceal the toys.

If you have no sensory table or sensory box available, and water play is not possible where you work, consider using your own hands. The child and the therapist sit across from one another. The therapist secretly selects a toy and holds it in her hands. Her hands then hide under the table. The child reaches under the table and feels for the toy. The therapist continues to hold the toy while the child feels it. When the child has made a few guesses, or when he guesses correctly, the therapist releases the toy for the child to bring up and see. This very intimate hand-to-hand play often encourages much spontaneous dialogue as the guessing progresses.

Social Networking

On-line social networking is one of the buzzwords among young people today. As we go to print, Facebook and Twitter are the premiere social networking sites of the moment, and they are hugely popular among younger people. On-line social networking should be a topic of conversation in the therapy room — whether the client's parents allow it, what type they use, how it works, and so forth. The process of using these forums can be discussed without computers in the room, or computers can be used to explore these topics together. For example, visit the client's Facebook page and explore it for the client's target phonemes. Be careful with all of this. Social networking sites are not filtered, and inappropriate material can arise. Consider studying the client's Facebook page ahead of time, but then pretending you have never seen it when exploring together with the client.

Sound Jars

LeAnn Sipple has her clients and their parents make a *Sound Jar* for home carryover. The jar is marked with horizontal goal lines to show how much it is filled with beans. Three key words are selected. Every time the child uses one of those three words correctly in spontaneous speech, the parent puts a bean in the jar. When a line is reached, the child selects from a list of pre-selected rewards. Over time the children become their own monitors of this, and then they have to ask their parents to put a bean in for them. I like this activity for several reasons. First, it stimulates awareness and self-discrimination. Second, it's easy for the parents and can be done on a whim without sitting down at a table to do speech homework. Third, the number of words is restricted. And last but not least, the children will go out of their way to say their target words often so they can get more beans in the jar! Terri Jones does the same thing in the classroom by using cotton balls. The client gets a reward when the jar is filled. She brings peers into the activity by having them serve as listeners who are ready to catch the client saying his sound correctly so he can receive a cotton ball.

Speech Badges

I have never done this in therapy, but I think it is a terrific idea for carryover. It comes from Berry and Eisenson (1956). Clients wear badges that instruct others to ask them a question during spontaneous interactions. The question is designed to elicit a spontaneous utterance from the children that contains their target phoneme. For example, if the client is seven years old and he is working on his S, the card might read, "Ask me how old I am." When asked, the child will answer, "Seven." To make the card simpler, it simply might read, "How old are you?" That way other children simply have to read the card verbatim. Berry and Eisenson suggested giving a badge with a question to each child in the classroom so the child with speech impairment does not stand out.

Speech Celebration Party

This is a carryover activity that involves speech students and every other student in their classroom. It will take an entire term and will end in a speech celebration party. Early in the term, the SLP works in the classroom to lead an activity for the entire class. During this initial activity (which may take several visits), the therapist encourages each child to come up with their own goal for improving their speech. The therapist explains that she will host a speech party for the entire class when every student in the room reaches his goal! The class works together to cheer each other on. This activity dovetails nicely with a classroom project about setting and reaching goals, and it is an excellent way to bring speech work out into the open.

The title *Speech Party* is written on the top of a poster board. The children enrolled in therapy are encouraged to write goals about their sounds like, "I will talk to 10 teachers using correct S," or, "I will speak slowly when I answer 10 questions in class." The non-speech students write goals like, "I will look directly at the teacher when I ask 10 questions in class," or,

"I will practice using a microphone, and I will speak slowly and clearly when I introduce 'The Reptile Man' when he visits school this year." The SLP can write the goals on the board, or the students can write them on index cards that are taped to the board. Each child is given a card on which they write their goal. This goal is kept at their desk, or in their own school binder, and is used to keep track of how they are doing on their goal. [Alternative idea: Use a 3-ring binder to record all this. Store it in the classroom for the children to review as needed.]

The goals chosen by the students are fairly big ones that will take several months to accomplish. The speech-language pathologist helps the children write goals, taking care that they are reasonable and achievable. The therapist continues to visit the class all year long during which she leads activities in which the students talk about what parts of their goals they have accomplished. She helps them record their progress on the poster. For example, the child whose goal was to ask 10 questions may have asked five of them, and this would be recorded on the chart.

The party is thrown when all the children reach all their goals. This celebration can be anything suitable, like a cookies-and-punch party or a field trip to a recording studio. Some of the children's goals will be met quickly while others will take some time. Unreasonable goals may have to be adjusted during the process. The poster (or notebook) is kept for the next year's students to show them how the process works. Older speech students can be chosen to help the SLP with this activity in the next class.

Speech Star Necklaces

Shanna Hess uses *Speech Stars* for carryover work at home. Each student gets a star to decorate. The star is then attached to a string and they wear it like a necklace around the neck. The children are told that they are to use their speech sounds correctly during conversation when they are wearing their star. The speech star also goes home for the child to wear after the parents are contacted about it. Shanna has found that using the speech star takes off the pressure parents feel when they think that they have to monitor and correct their children constantly. The method puts the work on the star and restricts it to only the time when the star is being worn. Shanna suggested that other shapes that are specific to the target sound might be used. For example, use the shape of a kite for K, a table for T, or a rainbow for R.

Speech Tag

Bosley (1981) recommended teaching mothers to play a specialized game of tag for developing listening at home. In the game, the mother says the target sound, and the child respond to it. Sometimes the mother says the sound correctly, and other times she says it incorrectly. She imitates the child's error exactly if she can. If the mother says the sound correctly, the child waits. If she says it incorrectly, he tags her with a playful slap on the hand. If the child fails to catch the error she made, then she tags him. Score is kept to find the winner. Rolls can be reversed to make it a production game. This is a nice simple idea for auditory awareness and early production work.

Speech Ticket Contest

Eliza Pelletreau gives teachers *Speech Tickets* that they hand out to the speech students as rewards during class. The tickets say, "I caught _____ using their good sound(s) during _____." Children turn in tickets for tiny rewards, like one Starburst candy for one ticket. The receiving of tickets also becomes a little contest in small groups where the first student to turn in a certain number of tickets wins. Eliza counsels with teachers about this process and gives them a short written explanation. The information sheet says, "Your student _____ has been working very hard to achieve accurate production of _____. He/she is able to use this sound during all structured speech activities with me. We would like your support in helping _____ carryover this skill to spontaneous speaking situations in other settings. Please fill out the tickets to reflect when and where you have heard your student using their good sounds." Eliza also gives a number of tickets to the students themselves to hand out to other important adults at school and home.

Speech Tokens

Debbie Neal has a great idea for rewarding kids when they speak correct words to the therapist outside of the therapy room. She doles out *Speech Tokens* that she makes herself. She writes or types the phrase *Speech Token* all over a colorful piece of paper. Then she traces, cuts out, and laminates circles from the paper to be used as the tokens. She keeps some of the tokens with her at all times. When her speech students approach and speak with her outside of therapy sessions, she doles out a token if they speak with correct sounds. The student may receive several tokens if he stays with her and talks for a while. She makes sure to make appearances in the hall, cafeteria, and recess locations during the school day. Students trade in their tokens for prizes in her therapy room. Debbie reports that the students are very motivated by these tokens, and she finds them rushing up to her to speak with her outside of class. She also reports that others therapists have adopted this idea with success. I love this idea. Imagine your speech students waiting anxiously for you to make an appearance in the cafeteria so they can rush up and show off their speech!

Start the Day Right

Sheila Stull helps her clients start the day right with a list of sentences to practice at home. She sends home a piece of bright blue or pink paper on which is written 2-3 sentences that are constructed with 5-10 therapy words each. For example, an R-sentence might be, "Sharon wore a short purple skirt to church on Saturday afternoon." The sheet is posted to the refrigerator, and the student must rehearse the sentences every morning. Sheila reports that the activity takes the students less than two minutes to do and that it gives them an opportunity to start the day with good speech.

States and Capitals

Marybeth Shearron reminds us that memorizing the states and capitals is an activity that almost every school child must do, and this is an excellent time to incorporate articulation carryover work. Therapists work with classroom teachers to make sure everyone is pronouncing the names correctly, and special emphasis is placed on the speech students' carryover productions. Opportunity to work on memorized material comes from other subjects as well. For example, we can help the children in their pronunciation as they memorize times tables, the presidents, the opening paragraph of *The United States Constitution*, a famous speech, a scene from a play, the periodic table of elements, and so forth.

Stop Lights

Lindsey Baker makes stop lights for the generalization phase with younger children. She laminates a red, green, and yellow paper circle. She uses these to provide feedback to the children about the sounds they are using in conversation. She posts the green if they are using their sound correctly all the time, yellow if part of the time, and red if no time at all. She finds this to be an easy way to get parents and teachers involved because it requires them just to listen, and it puts the weight on the child to do the work. She says that teachers especially like this idea. Rewards are given for times when the green light stays on.

Tallying Targets

Many therapists wrote in about how they used tallying in therapy. Correct or incorrect responses are tallied, and praise is offered accordingly. Linda Groszyk submitted a very interesting way to tally data during reading activities. She has a client read a book aloud. As he reads he tallies the number of times his target appears on each page. Then he writes that number on a sticky-note that is fastened to the page. When the book is finished, there will be a sticky-note on each page, and a total number for the book can be obtained. Linda says that this activity super-charges the clients awareness of his target. Each page is read twice. The first reading is very slow because of all the tallying, but speed and fluency improves during the second. [Note: Our library friends would tell us to make sure that the sticky part of the note is sticking to the page margins, and not to the printed words. Sticky notes pull letters off pages after repeated use.]

Teacher Notes

Many therapists provide teachers with notes to help in carryover. June Schroeder makes notes for each client who needs help with carryover. The note has a large picture of lips and says, "Ask me to say _____ and _____ and _____." The blanks are filled in with target words. The page also might have a question that the child must answer using his target word or words. June has these sheets signed by the clients indicating that she talks about this with them first so they know what will be coming in the classroom.

Telephones and Walkie-Talkies

Children usually love to play with telephones and walkie-talkies, and these can be a wonderful addition to a carryover program. They are highly motivating. I use both toy and real telephones and walkie-talkies, and young children hardly seem to notice the difference. I also use my cell phone and my office phone together to do speech work. While in the same room, I call them, or they call me, and we do our speech work just as we normally would in the therapy room but over the phone. This is a way to make speech work more like real life conversations. You can sit in the therapy room together, or one of you can be in the hall or other room. Telephoning also can be done while the client is at home. This is an excellent maintenance activity to be done in order to wean the client away from therapy.

Very old articulation texts recommended using telephones to facilitate carryover. In fact, the earliest texts even discussed how to use the telephone operator (called *central*) to make a call: "First call central and then speak slowly and melodiously" (Scripture, 1912, p. 221). Anne

Kropf uses her office phone to let clients call a family member in order to tell the person what they are doing in speech class or to talk on another topic. Gretchen Bergen has students call one another during therapy and play out certain telephoning scenarios. They report a fire, make an appointment, inquire about a certain product, ask a friend about a homework assignment, and so forth.

Tell-Your-Parents Homework

Melanie Hostetter has created half-page *Tell Your Parents* homework sheets she sends home with the students for parent signatures. Each page has an assignment. For example:

- Tell your parents what happened after school today.
- Tell your parents what you read in school today.
- Tell your parents what happened at your school special today.
- Tell your parents what happened in your classroom today.
- Tell your parents what happened at recess today.
- Tell your parents what happened at lunch today.

The slip also has lines that the children use to rate their performance that says: I correctly produced my speech sound(s):

- During the entire activity.
- During most of the activity (1-3 errors).
- During some of the activity (4-8 errors).
- During very little of the activity (9+ errors).

Ten Steps Game

Esther Baxter submitted a very interesting carryover activity she calls the *Ten Steps Game.* After a therapy session, she walks the student back to class. Every ten steps they stop and review their speech targets. If the client does not maintain the target, they back up ten steps and try again. She reports that the children love this game, and they strive to make it back to class without having to back up even once. Once they arrive at the classroom door, the student demonstrates for his teacher what he can do if she has a free moment. This is an excellent way to bring the work literally outside of the therapy room and to keep teachers abreast of what's going on in the student's therapy program.

Three-Ring Binders

In writing about articulation correction in 1971, Powers wrote, "Speech workbooks are a highly effective device to enhance motivation" (Powers, 1971, p. 900). I had always thought that the speech workbook was an old-fashioned way of doing therapy, but I eventually tried it. I found that constructing a speech binder quickly became my most favorite and successful way of promoting carryover.

The three-ring speech binder is constructed with papers made in therapy. One or more papers are added almost every therapy session. The pages are dated and placed in order, so the binder becomes a permanent record of all that the client has accomplished throughout the course of treatment. I like to put the pages in from back to front, so when the binder is opened, the first pages shows the most recent material. The binder becomes a great way to review work, discuss progress, and plan for the future. The activities of the day are recorded in one way or another on a page during the course of the activities. There are charts of progress, lists of key words, lists of the people with whom the client will try his new skill, pictures drawn of difficult communication situations, book reports presented to the class, poems written together, and so forth.

The old-fashioned speech binder may seem like an outmoded and corny idea for speech correction, but in my experience the speech binder has been the key to carryover for many of my clients. The speech binder makes the abstract work of speech correction something concrete. It gives a physical form to the treatment process. The binder becomes a book that the client can share with mom, dad, siblings, grandparents, and others. It helps the child answer that recurring question "What did you do in speech today?" The speech binder also becomes a record of the client's progress of change. It can become one of the most important documents he makes during his childhood: "Make the speech book attractive with pictures, drawings, stickers, etc. Help the child feel it is a prized possession" (Bosley, 1981, p. 23).

The speech binder is a very practical idea for private therapy, when we can be assured that the binder will go home and then come back again most of the time. Adaptations for the public school environment must be made. In the schools, create an additional tabbed section in the child's regular three-ring school binder. Put pages in that are to be removed at home. The removed pages can be placed in another binder at home for permanent storage. If possible, make duplicate pages to use as a second set to keep at school. When duplication is impossible, the therapist can make a similar page to put in a binder in her room. Put pages of all the children's work into one binder. Searching for the right page that shows what they worked on the last time is an excellent way to begin a new session.

Time Challenge Game

Donna Ridley plays a game called *Time Challenge* for carryover. The task is for the children to take turns talking spontaneously for a few minutes. They are timed to see how long they can go without error. The time the child achieves is recorded. The one with the longest time wins. Multiple turns can be taken and the times added to get a final score. Times can be graphed to show how they increase over time.

Time Frames

Some therapists have advocated that time frames be established for correct speech outside of the therapy room. For example, a client might be expected to speak correctly with his new sound from 8:00 to 8:15 every day. Choosing a time that will work every day may be difficult for some clients because of their varying schedules, but it can be done. Older clients who keep to their own daily schedule on a paper calendar can post the time. Clients with cell phones and other electronic devices can set alarms to ring when the time comes. Time frames are an excellent way to carry speech skills outside of the therapy room. They allow clients a concentrated period to focus on the skill every day, and they allow them the freedom to make errors outside of the time frame. Time frames should be increased from once per day, to twice per day, and so on, over time.

Topical Demonstrations

Pamela Williams uses classroom topics to develop demonstrations the speech students can do in front of their peers. For example, she had her speech students make Fry Bread during Thanksgiving week. The students taught their class the preparing, cooking, and serving procedures as they prepared the bread in the classroom. They also discussed the history of the bread. The speech students practiced the presentation in therapy beforehand. Pamela reported that the activity was a huge success, and that many students and teachers asked for the recipe. This made the speech students feel popular and successful.

Variety Shows

Have the speech students organize and put on a variety show. The students will ask their friends and teachers to be a part of the performance which will showcase talents—dancing, drumming, singing, piano playing, and so forth. This type of activity might take an entire semester to arrange. Lists and time schedules can be made. Rehearsals can be held. Good speech at a conversational level will rule each aspect of this complex activity.

Video Games

The best way to handle video games for the promotion of carryover probably is to ask students to talk about their favorite games, either with or without the games present. Kids love these games, and some have their minds on them all the time. Instead of trying to ignore the games to which your client is all but addicted, invite these games into therapy. A child's video pursuits may be his greatest passion and you might be the only adult who is interested in hearing him talk about it. Let him. In fact, the client may be living a life where every other adult is trying to get him to stop using or talking about the games. Some children open up about their video games and want to talk about them more than other activities. Ask clients simple questions about how to play, how to advance, how far he's gotten, who else likes to play, how often he plays, what other games are just like it, who buys the games for him, whether his bothers and sisters play as well, whether his parents play, and so forth.

Voicemail Messages

Many therapists suggested having clients leave voicemail messages as a carryover activity. This is such a great idea because children love using phones and leaving phone messages. Leaving phone messages can be done in at least two different ways:

- CALL THE THERAPIST FROM HOME: Have the kids call their therapist from their own home to leave a voicemail message in the evening or on the weekend. The client can speak extemporaneously, or he can practice his assigned speech work. This activity assures that the children are thinking about speech and practicing at home.
- CALL HOME FROM THERAPY: Have the children call their own homes during a therapy session in order to leave a message that they can listen to when they get home later. Voicemail left on the home phone is a way to bring speech work directly into the home to share with family members. Clients also can leave the same or similar messages on

each individual family cell phone.

Weekend Contract Cards

Robin Chopskie uses cards as mini-contracts for weekends. The mini-contract is written on an index card that specifies the work to be done over the weekend. For example, the card might read, "I will use my sound at least three times." The communication partner at home initials the card when the client carries out the task. The card also has a space for comments or reflection. The students get a reward if the contract card is returned.

Weeklong Homework Assignments

Virginia Shawron submitted a nice list of homework assignments that can be done over a week. Each one starts out as follows: *This week, I will keep track of using my clear speech...*

- When I read three poems aloud to my family members.
- When I read three children's books aloud to a younger child.
- When I sing or speak at religious services.
- Every time I talk to one of my parents or family members.
- When I talk to three of my friends. I will ask them to listen to my sounds and ask them how I sounded.
- At all of my meal times. If I make a mistake, I will correct myself right away!
- Whenever I am riding in the car. Whatever conversations I have in the car, I will be sure to use my clear speech!
- Whenever I am talking on the phone. I will make three phone calls to someone and I will be sure to talk with my clearest speech.
- Whenever I am talking in my class to my teachers or friends, or when I am reading aloud.
- At any of my after school activities.

Weekly Quotas

Some old-time speech correctionists advocated the idea of achieving a weekly quota of words to be remembered and uttered correctly outside of the classroom. For example, if the client is working on S, his target word might be *please*, and he might be required to say it 21 times (or three times per day) during the next week. The client would be required to tally his productions to make sure he made his quota. Tracking weekly quotas is an excellent way to bring conscious awareness of correct speech production out of the therapy room, and it becomes a point of review in subsequent sessions. Tracking quotas must be done on the honor system, of course, and it would be easy for clients to cheat. But a client whose personality is achievement oriented will enjoy this activity and will be motivated to do it honestly. In fact, the client will probably tell you, "I wanted to cheat but I didn't!"

What did you do in speech today?

This activity is designed to help clients answer the persistent question, "What did you do in speech today?" The activity is to prepare the answer. I use my speech binders in this process, but other written means such as cards or e-mails could be employed as well. In using the binders, I write a page that summarizes our activities. We write, "What did you do in speech today?" as well as the date on the top of a paper that is put in the speech binder. Then we simply list the session's activities. Together the child and I generate the items for the list. I help write the list so that others can understand the activities, and I write them myself with young children. Here are some examples from a client who is working on K at the beginnings of words:

- I practiced car, coat, candy, cab, coo-coo, cap, cart, keep, kitten, and kite.
- We played a guessing game. I guessed which card was in an envelop that was in a mailbox. I guessed 6 out of 10! Miss Pam said I did a great job!
- I used a mirror to watch my tongue making K in the back.
- I ate a gummy bear and watched in the mirror while I was chewing.
- I played basketball and won the game!

The activities can be listed as they conclude, or the entire list can be generated at the end of the session as a way to review. If the items are listed at the end of therapy, they will be in random order, but the order doesn't matter. The purpose of the activity is for the children to use it for recall at home later. I usually train parents to ask their student this question after every session, and then to encourage someone else in the family to ask it later that evening. The list also can be pulled out when other relatives visit. Grandma may ask, "What are you doing in speech now?" Instead of the child shrugging his shoulders, the child can run off to get his speech binder for grandma, and he can use it to help him talk to her about it.

What's Wrong Pictures

Alice Lamoreaux reminds us that children love *What's Wrong* pictures and that these pictures make an excellent way to stimulate spontaneous speech for carryover. She keeps several books that contain this material in her therapy room. The students take turns finding something silly in the pictures and describing it using complete sentences and correct sound productions. These pictures often stimulate laughter and silliness, two profound elements of carryover stimulation. There are card sets of these types of pictures available commercially that are marketed for language therapy. My set is made of photographs that depict many silly pictures, like a man in a business suit standing in a pond while fishing.

Word Games

Most children love word games. Word games have been mentioned as an excellent way to stimulate spontaneous speech since the beginning of our profession and many therapists still use them today. Word games can be played in therapy, in the classroom, or at home. Most families have their own set of word games they play in the car, and therapists can learn about them by asking the kids to show them how to play. Any number of word games could be used. Scores can be kept or the games can be played just for fun. Here are some popular examples:

- I SPY: Therapists who submitted ideas for this chapter mentioned this old stand-by word game the most often. One person identifies an object or picture that can be seen in the environment and says, "I spy, with my little eye, something that starts with the letter

K … something that is blue … something that is tiny … something that we eat." The other person has to guess the object by asking, "Is it a ___?" The guessing continues, and more clues are given, until the correct object is identified.

- ASSOCIATIONS: Association games also are an excellent way to stimulate spontaneous speech targets. Say a word, and have the client say a word that is associated with that word, for example: Car/drive, Shoe/wear, Picnic/ants, or Tuesday/Wednesday. Extend the game to include phrases and sentences, for example: Car/Drive to school, Shoes/I wear them, Picnic/I went on one last summer, Tuesday/I have football practice on Tuesday.
- WORD CHAINS: This is a memory game. The first child says a word. The second child repeats the first word and adds another. The third child repeats the first two words and adds a third, and so forth. The game continues until someone cannot repeat the chain of words. Much hilarity ensues as words are forgotten and mixed up. This game often is played with a carrier phrase like, "I went to the store to buy some _____ and some _____ and some _____."
- BUILD A SENTENCE: The group builds a sentence one word at a time, with each member contributing one word per turn. The turns continue until the sentence seems complete or until it becomes so funny that they cannot go on any longer. For example, Child A says, "The." Child B says, "boat." Child C says, "went." Child D says, "off." Child E says, "every." And so the game continues to build a sentence. The sentence may end up being, "The boat went off every day at six o'clock because people like banana dog milkshakes." Much hilarity and spontaneous conversation ensues.
- PIG LATIN: Most readers will remember speaking in Pig Latin during their childhood. Pig Latin is a word game played in which the first phoneme (or cluster) of a word is transposed to the end of the word, and the syllable Ay is added after it. For example, *bird* is changed to "Ird-bay," and *chocolate* is changed to "Ocolate-Chay," and planet is changed to "Anet-Play." Bonnie Chappell has her clients learn to change words, phrases, sentences, and entire stories into Pig Latin as a carryover activity.
- LICENSE PLATE GAME: This is a car game. Children take turns making up phrases to accompany the letters and numbers found on license plates. For example, DTR 175 might translate into, "Don't try reading 175 books," or, "David timed Ron at 175."
- VEHICLE IDENTIFICATION GAME: This also is a car game, but this one is best played when there is a person knowledgeable about cars present. Take turns naming the make and model of cars. Identify the ones that have the client's target sounds.
- VEHICLE IDENTIFICATION SOUND GAME: Identify the make and model of a car first and then change the name to reflect the client's target sound. For example, identify a *Ford Fusion*, and then change the name to "Shord Shusion" if the client is working on Sh. Make it slightly more difficult by adding an adjective or two before the name. For example, a *red Ford Fusion* would become a "Shed Shord Shusion," an *old red Ford Fusion* would become a "Shold Shed Shord Shusion," and a *beautiful old red Ford Fusion* would become a 'Sheautiful Shold Shed Shord Shusion." These utterances quickly become tongue twisters.
- MISSING WORD GAME: One child makes up a sentence and leaves out a word. The next child repeats the sentence and fills in the word. Outrageous fill-in words make this very

fun. For example, the first child says, "I hope there is ____ in my soup." The other child repeats with his own fill-in word replacement and says, "I hope there is a shoe in my soup." Expect the potty words to enter this game as it gets more hilarious.

- RHYMING WORDS: One child says a word and the other child has to say a word that rhymes. The rhymes bounce back and forth until one person cannot think of another rhyme. Then another word is chosen to begin another string of rhymes.
- FIRST AND LAST: This is an activity for children who can spell. One child says a word and spells it. The next child has to say a second word that starts with the last letter of the previous word, and he has to spell it. For example, the first child might say, "Car, C-A-R." The second child then might say, "Robot, R-O-B-O-T." The third child then might say, "Top, T-O-P," and so it goes.
- FAMOUS PEOPLE: This is a game for older children and adults. One person names a famous person, for example, *John Wayne*. The next person has to name another famous person whose first name starts with the first letter of the last person's last name. In our example, that letter would be W, so the next person to be named might be *Willy Nelson*. And so the game goes from person to person. Any famous person can be used—musicians, artists, politicians, movie stars, and even cartoon characters. Rules can be predetermined for incorrect, incomplete, or duplicated answers.
- TELEPHONE: Here is another word game that is an old stand-by. One child whispers a phrase or a sentence, or tells a short amusing story, in the ear of a second child. The second child whispers it to the third, and so forth around the circle until it comes to the last child who says it out loud. The transfer of the message from one person to another should have caused changes in the statements by the time the message gets to the last person. This causes hilarity amongst the children.
- NAME GAME: The process of making up nonsense words became a national phenomenon in the pop song *The Name Game* (first recorded by Shirley Ellis in 1964). A song like this can be adapted to a client's target phoneme. Do you know it? Here are two verses to get you started, otherwise look this up on the Internet to find various explanations about how to do it:

Micah, Micah, bo-bicah,
Banana-fana fo-ficah,
Fee-fi-mo-icah.
Micah!

Shirley, Shirley bo-birley,
Banana-fana, fo-firley.
Fee-fi-mo-mirley.
Shirley!

- MOONTALK: Gerber (1973) recommended the use of nonsense words in an activity she called *Moontalk* in which nonsense words are used as real words within a story about an alien. The alien visits earth and names the things he sees. For example, in working on initial S, he calls a tree a *simpa*, he calls a barn a *sikasoo*, and he calls a house a *salen*. Moontalk is a way to encourage creative thinking for carryover.

Word Search and Crossword Puzzles

Children love word search activities, and these can make a wonderful way to work on spontaneous words and letter names. A word search activity usually is intended as a quiet time activity, however the process can be changed to make it be a very verbal activity in a small group. Give one child the grid of letters, and another child the list of words to be found. Let the child with the word list guide the child with the grid by saying things like, "Find a D... Okay, now see if you can find a D with an A next to it... Does it start a word...? No? Okay, find an A ..." Make it more exciting by giving a copy of the word lists to all the other members of the group. See who gives the best clues to help the searcher find the words. Very simple crossword puzzles can be modified in the same way for group work by giving one child the grid and the other children the clues.

Words They Own

Ann Roman submitted an idea she got for carryover from Professor Wayne Secord in a continuing education seminar. Give the client an index card on which he will record the words he can say correctly. These are words the client owns. The card is kept in the child's pocket and pulled out for practice several times per day. Ann reported that she has used the idea with several boys who liked it very much. I think this is a good idea because it reinforces the child's success, it promotes self-confidence, and it affords practice outside of the therapy room.

The Word on Blogs

Many speech-language pathologists are writing blogs on which they post ideas about all aspects of speech-language therapy. Many of these posts contain ideas for parents to stimulate speech-language skills at home, and some even include ideas specific to carryover. Several therapists sent in their blog addresses as a contribution to this book. However, blog sites are changed almost daily, and it is impossible for a printed book such as this to be current on their content. As a result, we made a decision not to include blog references in this publication. Individual therapists can do their own web searching for blogged carryover ideas. Search under *carryover articulation*. This topic search also will bring up new research articles on carryover. Also search for material under specific carryover ideas. For example, therapists will find a plethora of therapy material by searching under *Tongue Twisters, Word Games, Hidden Pictures*, and so forth.

YouTube Videos

On-line videos contain an amazing array of subjects, and children love to watch and talk about them. Some are informative, some are amazing, and some are hilarious! On-line videos are very short, and they make a wonderful center point of discussion. Make sure to screen these ahead of time to avoid inappropriate topics. Let kids refer you to the ones they love best. Talk about the videos themselves, or use them as a platform to speak on any number of other subjects. YouTube videos of people and actors demonstrating different ways that English is spoken around the world are especially fascinating.

*

Chapter 9 Summary

Games and Activities to Promote Carryover

- Carryover must not be left to chance.
- This final chapter presented a wide variety of games and activities for the stimulation of carryover in articulation and phonological therapy.
- Some carryover activities are very cognitive in nature, and other ideas are playful and fun.
- Some carryover activities are highly structured while others are unstructured.
- Consistent use of the client's target sounds in spontaneous conversation is the ultimate goal of carryover activities.
- The client's ultimate task in articulation therapy is to produce correct articulation while his mind is otherwise engaged.
- Research, clinical experience, and the needs of individual clients shape the carryover process.
- Carryover can be stimulated in the therapy session, in the classroom, at home, in the car, on field trips, and just about anywhere that sounds and words can be discussed.
- Common sense, working theories, creative drive, and natural teaching ability are behind all games and activities designed to stimulate carryover.
- Competitive games are useful in carryover because they start out slowly and gain speed and energy within the session, thus reinforcing the notion that increasing speed of production is that which ultimately facilitates carryover.
- Many carryover activities stimulate humor. Children who can hold their speech together while giggling and laughing may have reached the pinnacle of carryover success.
- No one method of carryover should be considered more valuable than any other.

Final Thoughts

Therapy is a creative process based upon scientific research. Therapists study research and they study their clients, and then they experiment with ideas to achieve certain results. Carryover is approached in a variety of ways, many of which have been described this book. Research, clinical experience, and the needs of individual clients shape the carryover process. In this view, no one method is considered any more valuable than any other. All methods have value and will help certain clients at certain points in their speech program. The speech-language pathologist's work is to stimulate carryover by matching the right client, to the right method, at the right time.

References

Akin, J. (1958) And *So We Speak: Voice and Articulation*. Englewood Cliffs: Prentice-Hall.

ASHA/American Speech-Language-Hearing Association (2010) Evidence-Based Practice. *www.asha.org*.

Bankson, N. W. and Byrne, M. C. (1972) The effect of a timed correct sound production task on carryover. *Journal Speech and Hearing Research, 15*, p. 160–168.

Bernthal, J. E., and Bankson, N. W. (2004). *Articulation and Phonological Disorders*. Boston: Pearson.

Berry, M. F., and Eisenson, J. (1956) *Speech Disorders: Principles and Practices of Therapy.* NY: Appleton-Century-Crofts.

Blanton, M. G., and Blanton, S. (1919) *Speech Training for Children: The Hygiene of Speech.* NY: The Century Co.

Blockcolsky, V. D., and Frazer, J. M., and Frazer, D. H. (1987) *40,000 Selected Words: Organized by Letter, Sound, and Syllable*. Tucson: Communication Skill Builders.

Borden, R. C., and Busse, A. C. (1925) *Speech Correction*. New York: Crofts.

Bosley, E. C. (1981) *Techniques for Articulatory Disorders*. Springfield: Charles C. Thomas.

Brown, C. (1954) *My Left Foot*. Great Britain: Cox and Wyman.

Carrell, J. A. (1968) *Disorders of Articulation*. Englewood Cliffs: Prentice-Hall.

Carrier, J. K. (1970) A program of articulation therapy administered by mothers. *Journal of Speech and Hearing Disorders, 35*, p. 344–353.

Costello, J. and Bosler, S. (1976) Generalization and articulation instruction. *Journal of Speech and Hearing Disorders, 41*, p. 359–373.

Costello, J. and Onstine, J. M. (1976) The modification of multiple articulation errors based on distinctive feature theory. *Journal of Speech and Hearing Disorders, 41*, p. 199–215.

Diedrich, W. M. (1971) Procedures for counting and charting a target phoneme. *Language, Speech, and Hearing Services in the Schools, 2*, p. 18–32.

Diedrich, W. M. and Bangert, J. (1976) Training speech clinicians in recording and analysis of articulatory behavior. Washington, D.C.: US Office of Education Grant No. OEG-0-70-1689 and OEG-0-71-1689. [Cited in Bernthal and Bankson, 2004, p. 289]

Diedrich, W. M. and Bangert, J. (1980) *Articulation Learning*. Houston: College Hill Press.

Dinnsen, D. A., and Chin, S. B., and Elbert, M., and Powell, T. W. (1990) Some constraints on functionally disordered phonologies: Phonetic inventories and phonotactics. *Journal of Speech and Hearing Research, 33*, p. 28–37.

Dinnsen, D., and Elbert, M. (1984) On the relationship between phonology and learning. In M. Elbert, D. A. Dinnsen, and G. Weissmer (Eds.), *Phonological Theory and the Misarticulating Child*, ASHA Monograph No. 22, pp. 59-68. Rockville, MD: American Speech-Language-Hearing Association.

Dunn, C., and Till, J. A. (1982) Morphophonemic rule learning in normal and articulation-disordered children. *Journal of Speech and Hearing Research, 25*, p. 322–333.

Eisenson, J., and Ogilvie, M. (1965) *Speech Correction in the Schools.* New York: MacMillan.

Elbert, M., Dinneson, D. A., and Powell, T. W. (1984) On the prediction of phonologic generalization learning patterns. *Journal of Speech and Hearing Disorders, 49*, p. 309–317.

Elbert, M., and Dinnsen, D. A., Swartzlander, P., and Chin, S. B. (1990) Generalization to conversational speech. *Journal of Speech and Hearing Disorders, 55*, p. 694–699.

Elbert, M. and Gierut, J. (1986) *Handbook of Clinical Phonology: Approaches to Assessment and Treatment.* San Diego: College-Hill Press.

Elbert, M., and McReynolds, L. V. (1975) Transfer of /r/ across contexts. *Journal of Speech and Hearing Disorders, 40*, p. 380–387.

Elbert, M., and McReynolds, L. V. (1978) An experimental analysis of misarticulating children's generalization. *Journal of Speech and Hearing Research, 21*, p. 136-150.

Elbert, M., and Powell, T. W., and Swartzlander, P. (1991) Toward a technology of generalization: How many exemplars are sufficient? *Journal of Speech and Hearing Research, 34*, p. 81–87.

Elbert, M., and Shelton, R. L., and Arndt, W. B. (1967) A task for evaluation of articulation change. 1. Development of methodology. *Journal of Speech and Hearing Research, 10*, p. 281–288.

Engel, D. C., and Brandriet, S. E., and Erickson, K. M., and Gronhovd, K. D., and Gunderson, G. D. (1966) Carryover. *Journal of Speech and Hearing Disorders, 31*, p. 227-233.

Engel, D. C., and Groth, L. R. (1976) Case studies of the effect on carry-over of reinforcing postarticulation responses based on feedback. *Language, Speech, and Hearing Services in the Schools, 7*, p. 93–101.

Ertmer, D. J., and Ertmer, P. A. (1998) Constructivist strategies in phonological intervention: Facilitating self-regulation for carryover. *Language, Speech and Hearing Services in the Schools, 29*, p. 67-75.

Eysenck, H. (1990). Biological dimensions of personality. In L. A. Pervin (Ed.), *Handbook of Personality: Theory and Research* (pp. 244–276). New York: Guilford.

Faber, A. and Mazlish, E. (1980) *How to Talk So Kids Will Listen and Listen So Kids Will Talk.* New York: Avon Books.

Fisher, H. B. (1966) *Improving Voice and Articulation.* New York: Houghton and Milton.

Fisher, H. B., and Logemann, J. (1971) *The Fisher-Logemann Test of Articulation.* Austin: Pro-Ed.

Fry, E. B., and Polk, J. K., and Fountoukidis, D. (1984) *The Reading Teacher's Book of Lists.* Englewood Cliffs: Prentice-Hall.

Gagnon, E. (2001) *Power Cards: Using Special Interests to Motivate Children and Youth With Asperger Syndrome and Autism*. Shawnee Mission, KS: Autism Asperger Publishing Co.

Garber, S. W., and Garber, M. D., and Spizman, R. F. (1990) *Good Behavior.* New York: Villard Books.

Gerber, A. (1973) *Goal: Carryover, An Articulation Manual and Program*. Philadelphia: Temple University Press.

Gierut, J. A. (1989) Maximum opposition approach to phonological treatment. *Journal of Speech and Hearing Disorders, 54*, p. 9–19

Gierut, J.A., and Elbert, M., and Dinnsen, D. A. (1987) A functional analysis of phonological knowledge and generalization learning in misarticulating children. *Journal of Speech and Hearing Research, 30*, p. 462–479.

Gierut, J. A., and Morrisette, M. L., and Hughes, M. T., and Rowland, S. (1996) Phonological treatment efficacy and developmental norms. *Language, Speech, and Hearing Services in the Schools, 27*, p. 215–230.

Gierut, J. A., and Morrisette, M. L., and Ziemer, S. M. (2010) Nonwords and generalization in children with phonological disorders. *American Journal of Speech Language Pathology, Papers in Press.*

Gray, S. I. and Shelton, R. L. (1992) Self-monitoring effects on articulation carryover in school-age children. *Language, Speech, and Hearing Services in the Schools, 23*, p. 334-342.

Hanson, M. L. (1983) *Articulation.* Philadelphia: W. B. Saunders.

Hazel, E. L. D. (1990) Peer-assisted peer carryover alternatives. *Language, Speech, and Hearing Services in the Schools, 21*, p. 185-187.

Hegde, M. N. (1998) *Treatment Procedures in Communication Disorders*. Austin: Pro-Ed.

Hodson, B. W., and Paden, E. P. (1983) *Targeting Intelligible Speech.* San Diego: College-Hill.

Hoffman, P. R., and Schuckers, G. H., and Daniloff, R. G. (1989) *Children's Phonetic Disorders: Theory and Treatment.* Boston: College-Hill.

Irwin, J. V., and Weston, A. J., and Griffith, F. A., and Rocconi, C. (1976) Phoneme acquisition using the paired-stimuli technique in the public school setting. *Language, Speech, and Hearing Services in the Schools, 7*, p. 220–229.

Jewell, E. J., & Abate, F. (2001). *The New Oxford American Dictionary.* NY: Oxford University.

Johnson, J. P. (1980) *Nature and Treatment of Articulation Disorders.* Springfield, IL: Charles C. Thomas.

Kamhi, A. G. (2006) Treatment decisions for children with speech-sound disorders. *Language, Speech, and Hearing Services in the Schools, 37*, p. 271–279.

Kamhi, A. G. (2000) Practice makes perfect: The incompatibility of practicing speech and meaningful communication. *Language, Speech, and Hearing Services in the Schools, 31*, p. 182–185.

Koegel, L. K., and Koegel, R. L., and Ingham, J. C. (1986) Programming rapid generalization of correct articulation through self-monitoring procedures. *Journal of Speech and Hearing Disorders, 51*, p. 24–32.

Koegel, R. L., and Koegel, L. K., and Ingham, J. C., and Van Voy, K. (1988) Within-clinic versus outside-of-clinic self-monitoring of articulation to promote carryover. *Journal of Speech and Hearing Disorders, 53*, p. 392–399.

Leonard, L. B., and Webb, C. E. (1971) An automated therapy program for articulatory correction. *Journal of Speech and Hearing Research, 14*, p. 338-344.

Marquardt, E. (1959) Carry-over with "Speech Pals." *Journal of Speech and Hearing Disorders, 24*, p. 154-157.

McLean, J. E. (1970) Extending stimulus control of phoneme articulation by operant techniques. In ASHA Monograph #14, p. 24-47.

McNutt, J. (1994) Generalization of /s/ from English to French as a result of phonological remediation. *Journal of Speech Pathology and Audiology/Revue d'orthophonic et d'audiologie, 18*, p. 109–114. [Cited in Bernthal and Bankson, 2004, p. 290.]

McReynolds, L. V. and Bennett, S. (1972) Distinctive feature generalization in articulation training. *Journal of Speech and Hearing Disorders, 37*, p. 462–470.

Miccio, A. W. and Ingrisano, D. R. (2000) The acquisition of fricatives and affricates: Evidence from a disordered phonological system. *American Journal of Speech Language Pathology, 9*, p. 214-229.

Monahan, D. (1986) Remediation of common phonological processes: Four case studies. *Language, Speech, and Hearing Services in the Schools, 17*, p. 199–206.

Mowrer, D. E., and Baker, R., and Shultz, R. (1968) *S-Programmed Articulation Control Kit.* Tempe, AZ: Educational Psychological Research Associates.

Nemoy, E. M., and Davis, S. F. (1937) *The Correction of Defective Consonant Sounds*. Magnolia, MA: Expression.

Oller, D. K. (1978) Infant vocalizations and the development of speech. *Allied Health and Behavioral Sciences Journal, 1* (4) p. 523-549.

Polson, J. (1980) A survey of carryover practices of public school clinicians in Oregon. Unpublished Master's Thesis. Portland State University, Portland, OR. [Cited in: Weiss, C. E., and Gordon, M. E., and Lillywhite, H. S. (1987) *Clinical Management of Articulation Disorders, Second Edition.* St. Louis: Mosby.]

Powell, J., and McReynolds, L. V. (1969) A procedure for testing position generalization from articulation training. *Journal of Speech and Hearing Research, 12*, p. 629–645.

Powell, T. W. (1991) Planning for phonological generalization: An approach to treatment target selection. *American Journal of Speech Language Pathology, 1*, p. 21-27.

Powell, T. W., and Elbert, M. (1984) Generalization following the remediation of early- and later-developing consonant clusters. *Journal of Speech and Hearing Disorders, 49*, P. 211-218.

Powell, T., and Elbert, M., and Dinnsen, D. A. (1991) Stimulability as a factor in the phonological generalization of misarticulating preschool children. *Journal of Speech and Hearing Research, 34*, p. 1318-1328.

Powers, M. H. (1971). Clinical and educational procedures in functional disorders of articulation. In L. E. Travis (Ed.), *Handbook of Speech Pathology and Audiology*. Englewood Cliffs: Prentice-Hall, p. 877-910.

Ray, J. (2002) Treating phonological disorders in a multilingual child: A case study. *American Journal of Speech Language Pathology, 11*, p. 305-315.

Raymore, S. and McLean, J. E. (1972) A clinical program of carry-over of articulation therapy with retarded children. In J. E. McLean, D. E. Yoder, and R. L. Schiefelbusch (Eds.) *Language Intervention with the Retarded.* Baltimore: University Park Press, p. 236-253.

Rockman, B., and Elbert, M. (1982) An experimental investigation of individual differences and generalization in articulation training. Unpublished manuscript. Bloomington, IN. [Cited in: Rockman, B. K., and Elbert, M. (1984) Generalization in articulation training. In *Treating Articulation Disorders: For Clinicians by Clinicians*, Harris Winitz (Ed.). Baltimore: University Park Press, p. 131-152.]

Rosenwinkel, P. (1976) *Phonologically-Based Therapy for Children with Multiple Misarticulations*. Unpublished master's thesis. Urbana: University of Illinois.

Ruscello, D. M. (1975) The importance of word position in articulation therapy. *Language, Speech, and Hearing Services in the Schools, 6*, p. 190–196.

Ruscello, D. M., and Shelton, R. L. (1979) Planning and self-assessment in articulatory training. *Journal of Speech and Hearing Disorders, 44*, p. 504-512.

Sackett, D. L., and Richardson, W.S., and Rosenberg, W., and Haynes, R.B. (1997) *Evidence-Based Medicine: How to Practice and Teach EBM.* Edinburgh: Churchill Livingstone.

Scripture, E. W. (1912) *Stuttering and Lisping.* NY: Macmillan.

Shriberg, L. D., and Kwiatkowski, J. (1987) A retrospective study of spontaneous generalization in speech-delayed children. *Language, Speech, and Hearing Services in the Schools, 18*, p. 144–157.

Shriberg, L. D., and Kwiatkowski, J. (1990) Self-monitoring and generalization in preschool speech-delayed children. *Language, Speech, and Hearing Services in the Schools, 21*, p. 157–170.

Sommers, R. K. (1962) Factors in the effectiveness of mothers trained to aid in speech correction. *Journal of Speech and Hearing Disorders, 27*, p. 178-186.

Sommers, R. K., and Leiss, R. H., and Fundrella, D., and Manning, W., and Johnson, R., and Oerther, P., and Sholly, R., and Siegel, M. (1970) Factors in the effectiveness of articulation therapy with educable retarded children. *Journal of Speech and Hearing Research, 13,* 2, p. 304-316.

Sommers, R. K., and Shilling, S. P., and Paul, C. D., and Copetas, F. G. and Bowser, D. C., and McClintock, C. J. (1959) Training parents of children with functional misarticulations. *Journal of Speech and Hearing Research, 2*, p. 258-265.

Tabor, T. A. and Hambrecht, G. (1997) A clinical-investigator attempts to facilitate carryover of /s/. *Language, Speech, and Hearing Services in the Schools, 28*, p. 181-183.

Van Riper, C. (1954, 1949, 1947, 1939) *Speech Correction: Principles and Methods*. NY: Prentice-Hall.

Van Riper, C. and Erickson, R. L. (1996) *Speech Correction: An Introduction to Speech Pathology and Audiology*. Boston: Allyn and Bacon.

Van Riper, C. and Irwin, J. (1958) *Voice and Articulation*. Englewood Cliffs: Prentice-Hall.

Walsh, G. (1939) *Sing Your Way to Better Speech.* NY: E. P. Dutton & Company.

Weaver-Spurlock, S. and Brasseur, J. (1988) The effects of simultaneous sound-position training on the generalization of [s]. *Language, Speech, and Hearing Services in the Schools, 19,* p. 259-271.

Weiner, F. (1981) Treatment of phonological disability using the method of meaningful minimal contrasts: Two case studies. *Journal of Speech and Hearing Disorders, 46*, p. 97-103.

Weiss, C. E., and Gordon, M. E., and Lillywhite, H. S. (1987) *Clinical Management of Articulatory Disorders, Second Edition*. Baltimore: Williams and Wilkins.

Williams, A. L. (1991) Generalization patterns associated with training least phonological knowledge. *Journal of Speech and Hearing Research, 34*, p. 722-733.

Wing, D. M. and Heimgartner, L. M. (1973) Articulation carryover procedure implemented by parents. *Language, Speech, and Hearing Services in the Schools, 4*, p. 182-195.

Winitz, H. (1975) *From Syllable to Conversation.* Baltimore: University Park Press.

Winitz, H., and Bellerose, B. (1963) Phoneme sound generalization as a function of phoneme similarity and verbal unit of test and training stimuli. *Journal of Speech and Hearing Research, 6*, p. 379–392.

Wolfe, V. I., and Blocker, S. D., and Prater, N. J. (1988) Articulatory generalization in two word-medial, ambisyllabic contexts. *Language, Speech, and Hearing Services in the Schools, 19*, p. 251–258.

Wright, V., and Shelton, R. L., and Arndt, W. B. (1969) A task for evaluation of articulation change. III. Imitative task scores compared with scores for more spontaneous tasks. *Journal of Speech and Hearing Research, 12*, p. 875–884.

Young, E. C. (1987) The effects of treatment on consonant cluster and weak syllable reduction processes in misarticulating children. *Language, Speech, and Hearing Services in the Schools, 18*, p. 23–33.

Zagar, L. L. and Locke, J. L. (1986) The psychological reality of phonetic features in children. *Language, Speech, and Hearing Services in the Schools, 17*, p. 56–62.

Zehel, Z., and Shelton, R. L., and Arndt, W. B., and Wright, V., and Elbert, M. (1972) Item context and /s/ phone articulation test results. *Journal of Speech and Hearing Research, 15*, p. 852-860.